D0767823

Raw To Radiant

Kim Cohen

Raw To Radiant

ISBN 978-1-84728-501-0

Second Edition, October 2006
Radiant Health Publishing
970-920-2142

Table of Contents

Acknowledgments i
Introduction iii
Statistics v
My Transition to Raw vii

Section I

Raw food diets defined 1
Cause of disease 3
What cooking does to foods 7
Detoxification 13
Germ theory 21
Meat eaters vs. vegetarians 25
Raw foods 29
Proof/support for eating raw 39
Raw food combining 43
Digestion & elimination 45
Diseases cured by raw foods 47
Vitamins & supplements 49
Enzymes 53
Eating out 57
Weight 61
Water 63
Lifestyle changes 67
Equipment 71

Section II

Raw integration 75
Drink your vegetables 75

Eat Meats Raw 78
Eat more sushi 78
Cut out refined sugars 82
Add Terramin clay 84
Eliminate processed foods 85
Drink Lemon/cider honey tea............................ 86
Add raw fats 86
Smoothies.. 86
Healthy snacks 87
Closing words.. 89

Section III

Recipes... 91
Basic Green Juice 91
Lemon - Cider Honey Tea/Drink.......................... 92
Rob's Lemonade 93
Tropical Smoothie... 93
Orange Smoothie.. 94
Wild Salmon & Shrimp Ceviche' 95
Filet Appetizer 96
Buffalo Tartar... 97
Kathleen's Meat Loaf... 98
Beginner Chicken.. 99
Avocado Custard 100
Peach Ice Cream 101
Banana Ginger Ice Cream.................................. 101
Natashia's Banana Cream Pie............................ 102
Coconut Balls 103

References 105
About the Author 109
Index 111

Acknowledgements

I would first like to thank Dr. Aajonus Vonderplanitz. I believe the work he has done is more important than any other ground breaking work that has been done in the health care field in decades. He has inspired me to study this subject in great depth and seek out truths that are not discussed by main stream media.

Next, I would like to thank my mother for instilling confidence and perseverance. These have been just two of her greatest gifts to me and for this I am grateful.

Thank you to Branden Cohen for leading me in the direction of alternative ways. I grew up with only conventional knowing and hadn't even heard of the words "alternative" or "organic" until our coming together...Thank you.

Last, but certainly not least, I want to thank my daughter Sedona, who is truly the love of my life and for whom I hope to be a positive influence and role model.

Introduction

The purpose of this book is to provide you with information on food, nutrition and wellness that is not readily spoken about or marketed by mainstream media. This is information regarding what we as a culture have done to create disease and slowly kill ourselves (although lately it seems we are doing it much more quickly).

I am not here to preach to you, but rather to heighten your awareness of what we are doing to create the diseases we live with and to provide you with an alternative to improving your physical well-being. It is to make you aware of the choices you make each day so that maybe you can change **one** thing. Bringing your awareness to what you are putting into your body will facilitate small changes now that may lead to bigger changes in the future. I ask you to have an open mind and think "out of the box" when reading this book. It has come to you because you are ready at some level for this information.

I will inform you of the choices you have when it comes to treating ailments; specifically, how raw foods support the detoxification and healing process in the body. I have done extensive research on the subject of food and its relationship to disease and treating disease. I believe it is possible to treat and heal virtually any ailment with diet only. There is a tremendous amount of information on this subject, with plenty of evidence to support my teachings. Visit my website at www.RawToRadiant.com for related products and links to other sites.

Section I of this book informs you of how raw meats, raw unpasteurized dairy products (including milk, cream, cheese, butter, kefir and yogurt) and other raw fats (such as raw eggs, coconut cream, coconut oil and raw avocados), raw fruits & vegetable juices, raw nuts/seeds and their oils can provide all of the vital nutrients needed for a long life of radiant health. This is not about a diet of soaking nuts and sprouting grains. I will provide you with just some of the evidence that man is a raw meat eating animal and how eating plenty of raw meats, fats, fruit and vegetables are what man needs to heal himself of disease. You will no longer fear diseases or growing older. You will look and feel younger and healthier. Your food addictions will gradually fade away, and you will be able to live your life with health and vitality.

Section II teaches you how to slowly transition these foods into your current diet and lifestyle. Change can be difficult, so I have provided **10 easy steps** to slowly integrate these raw, life giving foods into your current diet. It doesn't matter if you are currently a meat and potatoes eater, a vegetarian or eat fast food. I will take you step by step through the process of making healthier choices and you get to choose the pace that works best for you.

Section III provides you with recipes that will make it easy to transition these life-giving foods into your diet.

Our aging population is growing faster than ever before. Take control of your health. Free yourself of disease and slow down the aging process now!

Statistics

- 50% of American women today (1 in 2) will die of Heart Disease at some point in their life.

- Children as young as four years old are showing the beginning stages of Atherosclerosis. 65% of urban American children aged 12-14 have fatty streak lesions in their arteries. 8% have lesions typical of more advanced atherosclerosis.

- In 2005, 570,280 Americans died of the following cancers: Lung, Colon/Rectum, Breast, Brain, Pancreas, Prostate, Ovary, Liver, Leukemia and Non-Hodgkin's Lymphoma.

- In the United States in 2005, there were 1,372,910 new cases of the following cancers: lung/bronchus, Breast, Prostate, Colon/Rectum, Uterine, Urinary, Melanoma, Non-Hodgkin's Lymphoma, Ovary, Kidney/Renal, Thyroid, Leukemia, Pancreas, Oral cavity/Pharynx.

- 20.8 million adults & children in the United States have Diabetes. It has now reached epidemic proportions.

- 4.5 million Americans have Alzheimer's disease. The number of Americans with Alzheimer's has more than doubled since 1980. By 2050, the expected number of individuals with Alzheimer's could range from 11.3 million to 16 million......Alzheimer's Association.

- In the United States, 58 million Americans are overweight, 40 million are obese and 3 million are morbidly obese.

- Autism is the fastest growing developmental disability with a 10-17% annual growth. Chances of a child developing it are 1 in 166 births.

- Between 1 and 1.5 million Americans are autistic.

- In a growth comparison during the 1990's, the US population increased 13%, while autism increased 172%.

My Transition to Raw

I feel it is important to share my background and experiences that guided my transition to raw foods as my story is that of a very ordinary person in which most people can relate. I was born and raised in the Flint, Michigan area. The only child of a single mother, I spent the first six or seven years of my life primarily raised by my grandparents. My grandmother made home-cooked meals of meat and potatoes every night and lots of pies. Everything was cooked in bacon grease. In fact, there was always a tin can of it sitting on the stove, ready for the hot skillet. Junk food, as we know it, was just starting to make its way into our home and I was a big fan of processed cereals and Ding Dongs. At about age seven, I was old enough to live at home with my mom, but because she worked full time, I was a latch key kid. Most of my meals were either TV dinners cooked in aluminum; toaster or microwave meals (later on); or fast food...lots and lots of fast food. It was cheap and we didn't have much money.

I will leap ahead to college where my diet consisted mostly of canned Spaghetti O's, white bread and salads. I was a dancer and gymnast, modeled and competed in the "Miss America" scholarship pageants to earn money for my schooling. Keeping my weight down was crucial and a constant struggle. In fact, when I ate a cooked diet, I always felt bloated and was one of those people that had to work out several hours a day, nearly seven days a week to just maintain my weight. It seemed that along with exercise, my caloric intake had to be extremely low (500 – 600 calories a day) to lose just a few pounds.

When I graduated from college, I was hired by one of the largest pharmaceutical companies in the world to sell prescription pharmaceuticals and pediatric vaccinations. I was later recruited by numerous medical companies and transitioned into medical sales (as opposed to pharmaceutical sales) with again some of the largest companies in their industries. I sold bone growth stimulators, titanium and stainless steel rods/plates and screws for spinal reconstruction, knee braces and heart catheters. In fact, I spent nearly 15 years training and working in the field of western medicine.

In my mid-thirties, I married and had a daughter that was born with severe food allergies to dairy (so I thought), soy, corn, wheat and numerous other foods. I had a difficult time finding treats that tasted good and that she could eat, so I created a cookie company called *Idella's Natural Gourmet.* I produced gourmet organic cookies that were free of wheat, dairy, soy and corn. Shortly after, I began studying nutrition and the healing effects of raw foods on the body. During my studies, I learned how ailments as we know them are really forms of detoxification. Stopping that detoxification process only pushes the toxins back into the system to restore.

While studying the health benefits of raw foods, I learned about the toxic effects of cooked foods on the body which meant I would have a decision to make. How could I continue selling (and making money from) my cookies, knowing they were contributing to disease in the human body? I couldn't, so I closed the doors of *Idella's* and pursued a career in nutrition, specializing in raw foods.

Dr. Aajonus Vondreplanitz was one of the many raw foods experts I studied. In my opinion, his work is the most important modern day work on the health benefits of raw foods. I refer to him throughout this book. When I first read his books, my initial reaction was that he was crazy, but there was something about the basic teachings that felt right on. I find it curious that humans are the only living creatures that cook their foods. It also seems so logical that we were created to eat food in its most natural state...raw and unprocessed. Because I was raised conventionally and with a background in western medicine, I needed proof. So, I have spent the past several years researching the teachings of Dr. Vonderplanitz and have found scientific evidence in support of them.

It took me several years to transition to a diet of 100% raw foods. In the beginning, the idea of eating raw meats was completely repulsive to me, especially chicken. In fact, it took me three years of eating raw meats before I would even taste raw chicken. I have learned that there are incredible dishes that can be made with raw meats such as Wild Salmon and Shrimp Ceviche' made with a red onion, jalapeno, tomato, avocado and cilantro sauce. The foods on this diet are incredibly appealing and take no time at all to make. There is an extra bonus as well, no messy cookware to clean up.

This is not a vegan diet of sprouting, soaking and dehydrating or trying to make nuts appear as some other food such as pizza. This is about eating what humans were designed to eat: raw meats, raw dairy, raw fats, raw fruit/vegetable juices and some raw nuts and their oils.

This diet has changed my life personally. I easily maintain a healthy fit weight; I do not fear eating fat and I do not fear disease any more. I am removing toxins from my body at an incredible rate and building new stronger cells in my body as well. You will read about Iridology and how the iris's reflect disease in the body. Take a look at my website www.RawToRadiant.com to see the color change that has happened in my own eyes. Look at the overall brown discoloration that covers my eyes in the first photo, then look at how the overall brown is disappearing and there is green and even blue showing through now. Filaments that were broken, thin and weak are now beginning to thicken, reattach and becoming stronger.

A few years before writing this book, I had over 12 hard lumps in lymph nodes all over my body that medical doctors could not diagnose. After only two years on the diet, all of the hard nodes had dissolved and softened. I have no doubt that I was on my way to Lymphoma.

Last winter every one of the 40 children of the two kindergarten classes where my daughter attends school were out of school for at least one - two weeks due to illness...except for my daughter. I know that her diet of about 50% raw, including a quart of raw milk every day, protected her. When she does begin the early stages of a fever, she knows that the house rule is...100% raw until we are healthy again. Along with much rest, I make a special orange smoothie at the onset of any illness and she is usually back to health within 24 hours.

I feel grateful and privileged to have had this information come to me and now I am able to pass it on to you. Eat raw and live!

Section I

Raw Food Diets Defined

First, let me define what raw foods are. They are all foods that have not had any kind of heat applied to them. They are foods in their natural raw form, the way nature provides them to us. Applying heat, even from a dehydrator, can destroy nutrients in food.

There are basically two types of raw food diets: One is a vegan raw diet where all of the foods eaten are fruits, vegetables and nuts. The other type of raw food diet includes raw fruits, vegetables and nuts, but also includes raw meats, raw eggs and raw unpasteurized dairy products. The vast majority of raw food eaters are vegan raw with some eating an occasional egg or piece of fish now and then.

This book will cover the importance of including raw meats, raw eggs and raw unpasteurized dairy products (including milk, cream, cheese, butter, kefir and yogurt) into a raw foods diet. As you will learn in later chapters, significant amounts of raw animal proteins and raw fats are crucial for vibrant health in the human body.

Cause of Diseases

When I first began to study nutrition, I was exposed to only the mainstream, conventional information that we have all heard at least bits and pieces of: Information like the importance of vitamins, a balanced diet according to the food pyramid and how it is necessary to steer clear of bacteria. As the years went on, I gradually uncovered the superficial information that had been sold to us to find deep truths about the foods we eat and their effects on our body.

I first want to talk about disease and where it stems from. Disease *(dis-ease)* is an imbalance in the body. The imbalance stems from two things: Toxemia & Malnutrition.

Toxemia is caused by toxins that enter the body in several ways. One way is through our environment. There is no denying that we live in a highly toxic culture and everyone is exposed to some level of toxins on a daily basis, especially in our industrial western culture. They are in our food, air, water, soil, medications and vaccinations. A second way toxins enter our body is by cooking the foods we ingest. I am here to tell you that cooking foods can produce toxic residues (mutagens) that accumulate throughout our body. We cannot escape toxins, but we can control the intake to a certain extent.

In 1980, The National Cancer Institute (NCI) hired The National Research Council (NRC) to study the relationship of diet and nutrition to cancer. The results were published in a book called, *"Diet, Nutrition and Cancer"*. They concluded that "chemicals found to alter DNA and cause mutations, have a high probability and should be suspected of causing cancer." They found mutagens in cooked meats and cooked carbohydrates, as well as coffee, tea, cocoa, red wine and grape juice (which are also all cooked or pasteurized). They found NO MUTAGENS in eggs, milk, cheese, meats and tofu UNLESS THEY HAD BEEN COOKED. If this isn't proof that cooking kills, I don't know what is.

A third form of toxicity is mental and emotional toxicity. I believe in the mind body connection and destructive thinking can poison the human body just as much as the toxic chemicals we ingest.

Nutritional deficiencies only add to the cellular breakdown going on inside of us. The standard American diet (SAD) is so void of nutrients that our bodies are breaking down at the cellular level. We are literally dying a slow death of malnutrition. Americans have an abundance of food to eat, yet the foods have almost no nutritional value at all. Biochemist, Harold N. Simpson, calls it "starvation in America".

The combination of toxemia and nutritional deficiencies causes Deoxy-Nucleic Acid (DNA) to mutate inside of us and we pass those DNA to our children. Our children continue to eat the cooked and processed foods that leave toxic residues in their bodies and are exposed to additional environmental toxins. Their DNA mutates even more and they pass these genes to their children. Do you see the pattern? What are we creating? This destruction and mutation is not always obvious for a few generations. The first one or two generations may not physically see or feel it, but eventually someone will have to live with the consequences. It is no wonder that children are born today with devastating diseases and that adults are plagued with chronic conditions developing so early in life.

I will give you another example of how toxins are passed from generation to generation. I have the lungs of a smoker and my daughter has smoking tars stored throughout her body, yet I never smoked, nor did my mother. But my maternal grandparents' chain smoked and those smoking tars were passed to my mother. She accumulated more smoking tars by growing up around the secondhand smoke and passed the smoking tars to me. I was exposed to the secondhand smoke for the first six years of my life and passed the smoking tars to my daughter. Imagine what my daughters' lungs would be like if both my mother and I had smoked? She may have been born with asthma or lung cancer.

The medical community does nothing to address this issue. It's only focus is on treating symptoms through drug therapy without enough research on the causes of disease. This is what physicians are trained to do in medical school, and what pharmaceutical reps are trained to teach physicians. Physicians learn a great deal from pharmaceutical reps. I know this because I was a top rep for one of the largest pharmaceutical companies in the world right out of college. Don't get me wrong, I have great appreciation for physicians that can save a life in the emergency room, or put broken bones back together, or reconstruct someone's disfigured face. But the bulk of medicine is managing chronic disease (which we have created) through drug therapy. We do not get disease because our bodies are void of antibiotics, sleeping pills, cholesterol lowering agents, weight loss drugs and pain medications.

One of the original founders of the Food and Drug Administration, Dr. Harvey Wiley, spoke of how the ingredients of cold and cough remedies all contain poisons that relieve conditions by suppressing the "detoxification process", thereby pushing all of the toxins trying to get out back into the body and adding additional drug poisons. Dr. Wiley was later forced from his position at the FDA because of his great knowledge on the natural healing effects of the body and the poisonous effects of pharmaceuticals.

The amazing thing is that the body will do its job if given the right tools. Its job is detoxification and healing, and the tools are raw foods, exercise, rest and a positive attitude.

"Thy food shall be thy remedy"- Hippocrates

Truly nutritional foods are in their purest form...RAW! Raw foods are what nature gives us to detoxify and feed our cells. A food in its purest raw form is loaded with all of the vitamins, minerals, enzymes, phytonutrients, amino acids and other nutrients that we don't even know about, but need to stay healthy. Cooking, freezing, pasteurizing, mechanically dehydrating and processing foods destroy the life in that food. Then, we put that dead food into our bodies and create toxemia (disease). Cultures that eat foods in their purest raw form have no degenerative diseases and live long lives of vitality. The wealthiest and most industrialized cultures (with the United States leading the way) have some of the highest rates of degenerative disease.

The next time you walk through a grocery store, really look at what is "alive" in the store....not much. Only "live" foods can be found around the perimeter of the store. The vast majority of foods found in grocery stores (even health food stores) are dead, processed foods. Nearly everything in the center sections of the store are dead foods and are the majority of what we are putting into our bodies.

Cooking kills...the food and eventually us. Life begets life!

What Cooking Does to Food

Destroying nutrients in food affect that food's assimilation in the body as well as causes toxic residues that store there.

Fats:
Heated fats, especially nut, seed and vegetable oils, are thought to be one of the worst things we can put into our bodies. This is because heating fats over 96 degrees F produce lipid peroxides which are carcinogenic. When fats are heated, they cannot exchange molecules correctly, causing them to dry out and harden. Therefore, they harden throughout the body such as in the arteries, lymphatic system and nerve endings in the brain. Cooked fats also cause osteoporosis and brittle bones as proven by the works of Dr. Frances Pottenger. Today, half of all women will die of heart disease at some point in their life (that is one of every two women you know). Cooked fats, especially cooked vegetable, nut and seed oils are one of the major causes of stenosis, hardening and plaque build up in the body. In general, women are smaller and would therefore have smaller arteries than men, so it doesn't take as much cooked vegetable oil, fat and cholesterol to harden and store as it does in men. Heart disease was not an issue before cooking.

You may be eating cooked fats that you don't even know about. All dairy sold in main stream stores in our country is pasteurized. There are only a few states in the country that have approved the sale of "raw" unpasteurized dairy in stores. In pasteurized dairy, the temperatures reach over 140 degrees F to kill everything in it. That means every life-supporting nutrient is destroyed as well. Synthetic vitamins are then put back into the dairy products so the labels can read "full of vitamins A & D". My daughter was born allergic to dairy (so I thought). I later found out that it was not the dairy she was allergic to, it was a combination of the added synthetic vitamins and lack of digestive enzymes (caused by the pasteurization process) that lead to her dairy intolerance. Since I put her on raw, unpasteurized milk she has had no problems at all. I believe that nearly all people that think they have a dairy intolerance do not actually have one. They are intolerant to the pasteurized dairy that is void of digestive enzymes and may also be intolerant to the synthetic vitamins added. All forms of dairy such as milk, cheese, butter, cream, yogurt and kefir sold in stores is made from pasteurized milk.

Edible oils are another fat you may think you are eating unheated. There are two primary ways of making edible oils. The first is through expeller (mechanical) pressing and the second way is through solvent extraction. Expeller pressing starts out with nutrient rich, healthy, life giving seeds that are mechanically cleaned and hulled and sometimes mashed. They are then cooked for up to two hours in various temperatures averaging around 248 degrees F. The cooked seeds are then pressed in an expeller press that also creates heat (through friction) of up to 203 degrees F. The result is a mechanically pressed "unrefined" oil. The second method of removing oil from seed is by solvent extraction. Seeds are ground into meal and mixed with a solvent such as hexane or heptane (also know as gasoline). The oil and solvent mixture are then separated from the seed and the solvent is evaporated from the oil at temperatures around 302 degrees F. This widely used method produces the highest oil yields and can leave residual toxic solvents in the oils. Some oils sold under the label as "unrefined" are mixtures of expeller pressed and solvent extracted. Refined oils are commonly taken through even more steps such as degumming, bleaching, and deodorizing. Though it may be hard to believe, the term "cold pressed" that is seen on so many labels truly means nothing!   There are no regulations set up for the use of these words. Oils that are put through an expeller press can still be, and usually are, labeled "cold pressed".

Heart disease and other degenerative diseases have been on the rise at an astounding rate since people have transitioned from raw butter to today's cooked vegetable oils. I truly believe these oils are one of our biggest killers. We are told not to eat saturated fats because they cause disease, and they do when they are cooked. Raw saturated fats do not as you will see in the chapter on raw foods.

Carbohydrates:
Cooked carbohydrates produce mutagens that store in the body.   The NRC publication, *"Diet, Nutrition and Cancer"*, reported that "the frying of potatoes and the toasting of bread result in the formation of mutagenic activity".   A study at Columbia University showed how cooking carbohydrates such as breads, crackers, pasta, cakes, cookies and other products from grains, produced something called Advanced Glycation End Products or glycotoxins. 70% of these toxins store in a healthy person and 90% store in an unhealthy person.   Stockholm University showed that cooking carbohydrates like French fries, potato chips, cakes, and bread, produce something called acrylamides that are known carcinogens.   The British Foods Standard confirmed the study, adding that acrylamides cause gene mutations leading to cancers including: breast, uterine and scrotum.   Dictionary.com defines an acrylamide as: "a white crystalline amide of propenoic acid can damage the nervous system and is carcinogenic in laboratory animals".   California has apparently passed a law where this information needs to be disclosed because I have stayed at two very popular California hotels that have this information prominently displayed. In one of the hotels, their room service menu states that they "serve foods that contain acrylamides which are known to cause

cancer". The second hotel has a plaque right at the front of the hotel when you walk in, as well as a plaque at the pool that also states that they "serve foods that contain acrylamides which are known to cause cancer." If this kind of disclosure were required throughout the country, every facility that served foods (including hospitals which are supposed to make us better) would have to have one of these plaques disclosing the truth.

Animal Protein/Meats:
Cooking animal proteins such as steak, chicken and fish, change the chemical make up of that meat protein. Scientists have been studying a group of known carcinogens called heterocyclic amines (or HCAs) which are formed when we cook meat. The longer meat is cooked and the higher the temperatures of cooking, the higher the rate of HCAs (these cancer causing agents). An article in *Environmental Health Perspectives*, entitled, *Heterocyclic Amines: Occurrence and Prevention in Cooked Food*, quotes, "Once metabolically activated, certain heterocyclic amines are among some of the most powerful mutagenic agents that have been detected up until now..." Thus, cooking meat forms HCAs which cause cancer! Another interesting finding is that the less fat on the meat, the higher the rate of HCAs. This means that those eating a grilled chicken breast have a higher risk of cancer from HCAs than those eating a rare fatty burger. All cooked meats have some level of HCAs, whereas raw meats contain no HCAs and thus do not pose a risk for cancer.

The NRC, when studying diet as it relates to cancer found that cooking beef stock in temperatures as low as 154 degrees F (less than boiling point), frying fish and broiling hamburgers, all produced mutagens. Again, mutagens are believed to be, even by the NRC, know carcinogens. We live in such a bacteria, viral and parasite phobic culture that we are doing everything we can to destroy them; and in the process, destroy the life giving nutrients in our food, as well as creating toxic substances that store in the body.

Fruits/Vegetables:
The cooking of fruits and vegetables destroys vital nutrients. Every cell in our body depends on nutrients for survival. The slightest destruction to these nutrients can affect digestion and absorption in the body. When these cooked foods are ingested, it causes nutrients to be leeched out of our body such as our skin, bones and other organs. (To understand more about how this process takes place, read the chapter on vitamins and supplements). Worse yet are canned or jarred foods. These foods are made with rotten and overly cooked fruits and vegetables that have no life in them at all...thus no nutritional value. In fact, the enzymes are often cooked out of the fruits and vegetables in order to preserve the color of the food.

The latest buzz word today is "phytonutrients". These are found in the skins of mostly fruits and vegetables and are in fact what give them their pigmentation (or color). Studies are showing their beneficial factors in enhancing the immune system and possibly preventing some forms of cancer. When scientists discover a certain phytonutrient from a particular food, it is assumed that all forms of that food contains the beneficial phytonutrient...this is not the case. Grapes for example, contain Flavonoids that carry many health benefits. It does not mean that red wine and grape juices also carry those same benefits. Both are usually pasteurized at temperatures of over 140 degrees F. As I mentioned before, this destroys vital nutrients including the health benefits of phytonutrients. The only way to get these phytonutrients is to eat the raw grapes themselves.

Detoxification

As I discussed earlier, disease is caused by both *nutritional deficiencies* and *toxemia* from volatile toxins in our environment as well as volatile toxins that are created when we cook foods. The removal of these stored toxins is crucial to staying healthy. Our bodies will naturally eliminate some of these toxins on its own but other deeply embedded toxins need to be helped along. In fact, there is no way our bodies can naturally eliminate the amount of toxins we are bombarded with on a daily basis without help. Everything that is excreted from our body has the potential to carry toxins out. Fecal matter, sweat, saliva, breath, mucus, ear wax, tears, vaginal discharge, skin eruptions and vomit are all modes of transportation for toxins out of the body. There are specific foods that can assist the body in ridding itself of toxins as well.

Let's discuss childhood illness as it relates to detoxification for a moment. We all know that pediatricians' offices are jammed with what we call "sick" children. They have runny noses, watery eyes, fever, cough, phlegm, diarrhea, rashes, and the list goes on and on. These children have come into the world (and ultimately the doctor's office) full of toxic waste and their bodies are doing everything they can to eliminate that waste. Today's mothers' bodies are generally not a healthy environment for a baby to grow. They are full of toxic residue from cooked foods, pharmaceuticals, alcohol, cigarettes and numerous environmental pollutants. When a baby is born, it is given formula, soy or rice milk, which causes additional toxic build up, or he is being nursed by a mother with the best of intentions but whose breast milk carries toxins in it. Now, I fully support nursing for as long as possible, I am just trying to give you an idea of where these toxic build ups come from in our children.

Henry Bieler, MD, in his book, "*Food is your best Medicine*" says, "The average baby comes into the world with his body full of toxins from the mother's blood and an intestine full of meconium. He is, in fact, so toxic that even with the best care it usually takes three years to eliminate his inherited birth poisons".

Since the book was written, here it is, 40 years later, and toxic levels in children are even higher and it takes even longer to rid those toxins from their bodies. This is why childhood diseases and ailments are so important. They are the detoxification process. Every ailment that a child experiences is nothing more than toxins trying to escape. Let the process do its work. Stopping a cold, flu, fever and all the symptoms only pushes the toxins back down to store and become something worse later on in life. In addition, giving medications only add to the toxic accumulation. Aspirin for example, deadens nerve endings, masking pain. Do you think aspirins long term effects on nerve endings are contributing to the neurological disorders of today?

Ian Sinclair, an Australian natural health researcher and author of "*Health: The Only Immunity*", describes how toxemia turns into disease. He describes how toxins enter the body, causing it to go into elimination mode that we call *acute disease* such as: cold, flu, chicken pox, skin rashes, tonsillitis, and other well known childhood diseases. When we suppress acute disease and their symptoms, we are suppressing detoxification and acute disease turns into *chronic disease:* arthritis, diabetes, ulcers, chronic fatigue, fibromyalgia, Alzheimer's, etc. When these continue to be suppressed with medications, diseases such as cancer have a greater chance of occurring.

"Cancer...and all chronic diseases were once innocent colds..."
- Dr. JH Tilden

When the body is detoxifying what has accumulated, the level of detoxification determines the label (ailment) the medical community gives it, such as a Cold, Flu, Tonsillitis or Cancer. When the body is not given enough of the essential nutrients for survival, diseases like Anemia, Osteoporosis, MS and Parkinson's Disease develop. In both instances, the body is telling you that attention needs to be brought to this matter.

Now, this part about detoxification may be new information and may be a bit shocking to most people. This is where you really need to think "outside of the box". Bacteria, viruses, parasites and mold all support the detoxification process. It has been proven that they breakdown unhealthy tissue from the body...and here's how. When a bacteria, virus, parasite or mold either enter the body or is created in the body, it feeds on degenerative tissue only, not healthy tissue. Think of how maggots or leeches (which are making a comeback in western medicine) work. They are put in a wound to clean up the garbage. They are the scavengers. When they are finished eating away the degenerative tissue, they drop off leaving healthy tissue behind. Bacteria, viruses, parasites and mold all do a similar thing inside the body. They are the garbage eaters of our bodies. We need them to break down degenerative or dead tissue in the body so we can eliminate it more efficiently. The key factor to getting healthy is what we ingest during and after this detoxification process.

Try to visualize bacteria that we have ingested eating away or breaking down degenerative tissues in the body. Now, if we continue putting cooked foods that create even more toxins into our body, we are giving that bacteria more to feed off of. If however, the bacteria is eating degenerative tissue and we are eating foods that actually regenerate new cells (like raw meats with raw fats), then we are getting healthier! This is why I am not afraid of eating raw meats and dairy. I am not afraid of bacteria anymore and trust me when I say, that was not always the case. I was one of those people who would clean my counters with the most powerful detergents after preparing chicken, then throw away the sponge for fear of the bacteria.

Sometimes when a person with a high inner toxicity level or a lot of degenerative tissue starts on a raw foods diet, they can go through an intense detoxification at first, whereas, someone with not as much accumulated toxicity or degenerative tissue may have no symptoms at all. To illustrate this, when I first started eating raw foods, I shared a piece of raw meat with a friend. I ate one or two small bites of the raw steak. He ate the entire remaining piece of a 24 ounce steak. I had diarrhea for three days while he had no visible reaction whatsoever. His body was relatively clean and the environment in my body was much more toxic. The bacteria had more degenerative tissue to feed off of. At the time, I was dumping toxins into my Gastrointestinal (GI) system and the bacteria had a lot of toxins to remove. Today, after being completely raw for many years now, I can eat "High Meat" (meat that has been aged a minimum of 2-3 months and allowed bacterial growth) and have no visible effects such as the diarrhea. And, I look and feel younger and healthier than ever.

Other examples of this bacterial and viral detoxification are being proven in medical universities all over the world.

- Swiss researchers injected colon cancer cells with a virus and eliminated the cancer. They noted that "viruses could damage cancer cells while sparing normal cells".

- Researchers from Stanford University, The Mayo Clinic in Rochester, MN and the M.D. Anderson Cancer Center in Houston injected the common cold virus into patients with gastrointestinal cancer that had spread to the liver. The patients tumors shrank and those receiving the highest dose of the virus lived the longest. They noted no risk besides having mild flu like symptoms.

- As reported in the New York Times, Dr. James Arseneau, at Albany Medical Center is testing the injection of a virus into advanced head and neck cancer patients with "superb results".

- A study published in *Nature Medicine* shows how a team at Harvard Medical School injected brain tumors with the herpes virus enabling the virus to destroy the tumors. Typically, most patients with *Glioma*, an aggressive form of brain tumor, die within one year. "This treatment is more effective than anything we have done before" says Antonio Chiocca, Harvard Medical School associate professor of surgery at Massachusetts General Hospital.

- Scientists from Calgary and London, Ontario have used a poxvirus to kill human brain tumors in mice. The poxvirus showed in the tumor but did not spread to other parts of the body. This study was published in the journal *Cancer Research*.

- Yale University proved that Salmonella bacterium reduced solid cancerous tumors in mice. Vion Pharmaceuticals is doing current testing on humans with a drug called Tapet that is an attenuated form of Salmonella because there is evidence that salmonella scavenges the body of degenerative and toxic tissue.

- Cultures all over the world eat salmonella on a regular basis to cleanse and detoxify.

It seems that in the not so distant future we will be paying pharmaceutical companies for bacteria and viruses to make us healthier. We do not need to pay for a bacteria or virus that was created in the lab when nature gives us everything we need. Bacteria and viruses come in contact with us on a daily basis. If the environment of our body needs that particular bacteria or virus to detoxify, it will use it. Let this process happen. I would rather live a life of an occasional detoxification in the form of a cold or flu now and then, than to have to go through radiation and chemotherapy or the injection of a virus into a cancerous tumor sooner or later in life.

How do you think man survived on farms not long ago eating the raw eggs right out from under the chickens and drinking the milk right from the cows? Studies have proven that children who grow up on farms around all of the animals and the bacteria and who drink the fresh "raw" unpasteurized milk are far healthier than children that do not grow up exposed to farm life. They are constantly touching animals and in contact with animal feces. In addition, they play in the dirt then touch their mouths, eyes and noses. Did you know that botulism lives in the dirt? Bacteria gets inside of them causing small continuous detoxifications which usually go unnoticed. We need these bacteria for our own survival.

When I eat out, nine times out of ten, it is sushi. Over and over again I hear sushi chefs, originally from Japan, describe how they grew up eating raw chicken, pork, beef and of course fish, as well as drinking fresh raw unpasteurized milk, eating raw unheated honey and raw eggs. They beg me for sources and information on how to get these healthy foods here in the United States. I believe the health industry has neglected studying the truth of why the Japanese lived longer until we brought in our Western eating habits. It is the raw meats, raw dairy products and raw eggs that have kept them so healthy for so many generations, not the soy. The western food industry has jumped on the soy "band wagon" which has been providing Americans with soy products that have been so processed that they don't even resemble food any more and are highly toxic to our systems.   The Japanese did not consume soy in this manner.

Humans, animals and plants, including bacteria, viruses, parasites and mold, were all put here to live harmoniously with one another. Think about how vegetation begins to deteriorate. A piece of fruit or a vegetable is plucked off of a plant when it is at it fullest life. If it is not eaten, it sits in our refrigerator or on our counter and begins to die. As it dies, it deteriorates and mold grows on it. The mold has a purpose, to break down the degenerative material.

Take two pieces of meat and put them out on a counter. Make one piece a freshly cut raw steak and the other a well cooked steak. Watch them and you will see that the cooked steak begins to mold and decay much faster than the raw steak. You may even see maggots appear on the cooked steak. That is because the cooked steak is dead and needs to be disposed of immediately. This is why bacteria grow on cooked meat much faster than on raw meat and why bacterial food poisoning is usually from cooked foods. Nature provides what is needed to assist in the decomposition process. The raw steak will take much longer to break down because it is still alive. As time goes by and that life decreases, it too will break down and need to be disposed of.

Nature works to break down degeneration with bacteria, viruses, parasites and mold. Then, our bodies work to eliminate that waste. Let it do what it was made to do. Don't stop the process.

I personally believe that one of the contributing factors to disease is that we are too clean. I will use bacteria phobia as an example. We are killing all of the tiny amounts of bacteria around us that are there to do their job...break down degeneration so the body can eliminate it easily. Because we live in a world where bacteria are all around us and we cannot escape it, we will eventually come in contact with it at some point. When we do, it will have so much built up degeneration to eliminate from our body that we will experience an intense cleansing and detoxification in the form of diarrhea, vomiting, fevers or what some may call "food poisoning". This is really nature trying to assist us in eliminating dead tissue so we can rebuild new healthy tissue.

Bacteria, viruses, parasites and mold break down toxicity and degeneration so the body can easily eliminate it.

Symptoms of detoxification should be called cures, not ailments! For example, a fever increases to speed up toxic waste removal; vomiting and diarrhea are the body's way of efficiently eliminating toxins; tiredness occurs so the person will rest and deep healing can occur; skin rashes are toxins being excreted through the skin.

Nature gives us what we need to take care of ourselves. So, when we get a cold or flu, be happy! Don't stop it from happening. Toxins are trying to escape from your body and stopping the detoxification process only pushes the toxins back down into the body to restore and become disease, possibly a very serious disease somewhere in the future. Medications stop the detoxification process from happening and store more toxins in the body.

Germ Theory

Louis Pasteur is best known for formulating the germ theory. His idea was that an outside organism (a germ) would enter a human body, reeking havoc on their system. He believed that these "germs" were monomorphic, meaning they have only one form and are non-changeable, although he was never able to prove his theory. There is much controversy written about Pasteur and his methods. It is said that many were not properly carried out and many more unscientific. For example, in one study, Pasteur injected the blood of one sick animal into a healthy animal making the animal sick. He concluded that the germ from the sick animal is what made the healthy animal ill. He forgot, however, to take into account what else may have been in that blood that may have contributed to the illness (more on this later).

Around the same time as Pasteur, a contemporary of his, Antoine Bechamp, was finding no truth to the germ theory in his research. In fact, he and many other colleagues were able to prove quite the opposite, that cells contained molecular granulations which he called "microzyma" and Gunther Enderlein called endobionts (Greek for bios-life). These microorganisms live inside us and cannot be destructed. They are pleomorphic, meaning they can change into many forms. It has been proven that they can enter four different stages at any given time. They can morph from a microbe to bacteria to a fungus to a virus. Dr. Robert Young, author of the book "*Sick and Tired*", has actually seen a red blood cell turn into a bacteria and then back into a red blood cell again. Dr. Aajonus

Vonderplanitz has proven through studies, that the body can create its own parasite as well. This may be a fifth stage of the morphing microorganisms. The microzyma or endobionts morph into whatever form the body needs to detoxify or break toxins and degeneration down.

These microzyma live inside every one of our bodies. They are virtually indestructible and they can change. The terrain or environment of the body determines what form they take. As talked about in the second chapter on the *Cause of Disease*, it is the lack of nutrients, as well as the toxins that enter the body, that alter its terrain or environment, causing the microzyma to morph into whichever form it needs for detoxification.

With Pasteur's study in which he injected the healthy animals with the blood of the sick animals, it was not the germ that caused the illness, but rather the toxins in the blood that were injected causing a detoxification in the healthy animal.

Dr. John Heritage, of the School of Biochemistry and Molecular Biology at the University of Leeds, wrote in his "*Notes on Microbial Infection for Medical Physicists*": "We are only 10% human. It has been estimated that there are about 10 to the 14th power cells in the human body. Of these, only 10% are of human origin. The remainder are the microbes that compromise our commensal flora. These are the microbes that live in and on our various body surfaces. We provide the microorganisms with food and shelter. In return, the commensal flora can play an important role in preventing infection. Without microbes, life on Earth would not exist. They are responsible, for example, for nutrient cycling. Certain bacteria, for example, are the only organisms that can fix the atmospheric nitrogen and make it available for other life forms, all which depend upon a steady supply of fixed nitrogen to survive". Wow!

I am not saying that it is not possible to obtain an outside organism, but one will not experience a detoxification or cleansing from it unless your body needs it (at least not a cleansing that is noticeable).   We all come in contact with hundreds, maybe thousands, of bacteria and organisms every day and yet we do not get sick every day.   That is why Pasteur's germ theory does not hold up.   Many people with a particular disease show no signs of having a specific germ that caused that disease.   And, many healthy individuals have shown signs of so called "pathogenic germs".

This is why I asked you to be open and think "outside of the box".   Louis Pasteur's unproven theories took off like wild fire. The important and proven works of Bechamp, Naessen and Enderlein were lost in the feeding frenzy of vaccinations, pharmaceuticals and the big business of the "germ theory". The health care industry's basis on the germ theory has created one of the biggest (if not the biggest) industries in the world. The mega food industry is right up there with it, due to the fact that what we ingest affects our health.   Money was, and still is, the motivating force.   Today's physicians are only preaching what they have been taught in school and hear in seminars.   As I said before, they do not know any different.   They are taught the theories of Pasteur and how to treat symptoms with pharmaceuticals.   I believe that they truly believe what they are doing is beneficial.   There are a very few around the world that are just beginning to have an open mind to the other concepts I discussed.

Every living thing has a way of cleaning up its own garbage. Watch a pile of compost decompose.   Mold, parasites and bacteria do their jobs to break down dead materials.   Mold, parasites, bacteria and viruses do the same thing in our body. They break down and eat up dead and toxic tissues so we can eliminate them more efficiently.   We have everything we need inside of us and all of the foods we need to support our health.

I watched an infomercial touting the effects of a colon cleansing supplement. The developer described how upon autopsy, colons have been discovered that were up to nine inches in diameter, impacted with fecal matter from toxic cooked foods and full of parasites. Now, the impacted fecal matter is due to the toxic diet of the individual, but the parasites are there for a reason, to clean up the impacted fecal matter.

Why then do we hear the occasional story of someone who supposedly contracted a deadly bacteria that was eating away at their body? Because that person had a tremendous amount of toxicity and degenerative tissue that needed to be broken down so the body could easily dispose of it. I believe that if they had eaten foods that were supportive to the body and were creating life in the body, they would not have had to go through this intense detoxification process. In addition, while in the detoxification process, they may have gotten healthier if they were on a raw foods diet that consisted of specific foods that would regenerate and rebuild new healthy cells.

If germs really made us sick then we would all be sick every day of our lives. We are in constant contact with millions of bacteria and viruses every day. Our body creates what is needed when it is needed. We are pumping ourselves with antibiotics that kill off helpful bacteria and bacteria are mutating to form strains that are resistant to these antibiotics, not so they can harm us, but so they can save us.

Note: Louis Pasteur himself apparently could not allow himself to die without the truth being told. On his death bed, he confessed that he believed it is the terrain, not the germ that causes disease.

Meat Eaters vs. Vegetarians

There is no doubt in my mind after researching this subject that humans are very much meat eaters. I have found so much Anthropological evidence to support this fact.

About four million years ago, the first humans (the Australopithecines) ate a large amount of small animals and were scavengers of the remains of large animals. They ate some plant foods, but their main source of nutrition was animal protein. Man evolved into Peking and Java man, Neanderthal man and Cro-Magnon man. As this evolution took place, man increased his ability to hunt and was able to capture and eat wild game. Although man was omnivorous, from the very beginning his diet relied heavily on meats.

It is thought that agriculture began about ten thousand years ago when wild game started to become exhausted. However, crops were not grown for eating. They were grown to begin raising domesticated animals for their meat. A bone found from a woman dating 5735-5630 BC, in the United Kingdom, proved "the woman's diet was virtually as meat-rich as that of a carnivorous wild animal". Near her thigh bone was found the bones of aurochs, deer and otter.

The Neolithic period, 4100-2000BC, has been associated as the period that farming began. Stable isotopes have been used to measure the amounts of bone protein in the bone of Britain's Neolithic man. The levels were sometimes higher than that of a carnivorous animal. These so called 'first farmers' were eating large amounts of meats, including animal products such as dairy.

As wild game became scarce, man settled down to raise domesticated animals for meat. There began the formation of organized religion. As this occurred, some religious groups gradually adopted "no meat" beliefs. Anthropologist Marvin Harris points out that Hindus were meat eaters before they converted to vegetarianism. And, the Dali Lama began eating animal meats after being advised by his physicians that he needed this to improve his health.

There is evidence that no ancient culture around the world has ever been totally vegetarian. Each has always had some sort of animal meat in its diet. Doctors Weston Price and Francis Pottenger traveled around the world in the 1930's and during this time, they could not find one long-lived society on our planet that was primarily vegetarian. On the contrary, there are numerous cultures that lived almost exclusively on meats and meat fats such as the Eskimos that were studied by anthropologist Vilhjalmur Stefansson, as well as many tribes in Africa.

In addition to this Anthropological evidence, we can take a look at how the intestines are designed in man versus animals that consume primarily vegetation. In a paper entitled "Can We Prevent and Cure Most Diseases by Nutrition?", written by D. Paul Cohen, president of the Cohen Independent Research Group, a Wall Street research firm, Dr. Aajonus Vonderplanitz, who was interviewed, describes how humans are not designed to digest raw whole vegetables and grains. He says, "Our intestine is 2 ½ times shorter than most herbivores (animals who mainly consume vegetation, such as cows, deer and sheep). We have only one stomach while herbivores have 2-4. Herbivores have nearly 60,000 times more enzymes than humans to disassemble cellulose (plant fiber) to obtain the fat and proteins from vegetation and grain. Vegetable fiber passes through an herbivores digestive system in about 48 hours. In humans, it passes through in 24 hours with only 1/3-1/2 of the cellulose digested, leaving most of the protein and fat undigested. Basically, we don't digest raw whole vegetables and grain well. We cannot utilize that which we cannot digest."

Notes on vegetables and vegetarians:

I have not updated the book recently but this section needs some clarification. I am not opposed to people being vegetarian if they do well on that kind of diet. But, there are some people who do not get enough protein on a vegetarian diet to rebuild new healthy cells as fast as they are detoxifying and thus need animal protein. This is actually the majority of the clients I have seen.

Also, I am not opposed to eating whole vegetables. It is just that many people cannot digest whole vegetation well in its raw form so juicing is best. The body does not have to break down and digest the cellulose. If eating whole vegetation (except for salads), I actually recommend the veggies are lightly steamed as this assists in digestion for most people. Some raw honey with the meal also aids in digestion.

Raw Foods

When I am speaking of eating raw, I am not talking about a life of salads, sprouting and dehydrating. I do not believe the human diet should be vegan or vegetarian or that we need to spend our time soaking sprouting or pulverizing nuts. My research proves that we are meat eaters and that our body needs animal proteins to live with radiant health. I have only ever met one raw vegan that did not look totally emaciated. In fact, there are vegan raw gurus that are searching for and creating protein powders (made mostly of nuts & seeds). They are trying to get more protein into their diets to increase size and strength and improve their health. Again, nature gives us what we need in animal proteins. The human body cannot digest huge amounts of nuts and seeds.

Food in its raw form has the perfect combination of nutrients and can be easily absorbed and assimilated in the body. Destruction of even just a few nutrients through cooking throws off the delicate natural balance of nutrients in that food. We have all heard the recent talk of how when we take one specific vitamin, others are necessary to make that vitamin work. Raw foods provide the exact balance of nutrients so that each nutrient can work synergistically with each other.

When eating raw foods, your body is constantly going through a detoxification process. In addition, if you are eating the proper foods for cellular regeneration, it is also going through a rebuilding process. This is the only way to true radiant health: detoxifying and rebuilding of the cells in the body. It is important to know this because every person's process is different. I have clients that feel great immediately after going raw and others that have taken 3 months, 6 months, or a year to really feel great. It is determined by how much and where the toxins have stored in your body and how intense your body is detoxifying at that moment. I personally went through an intense detoxification process the first 3 months of eating raw, then I felt great for 2 years following that and then went through another intense 6 months of off and on detoxification and healing. This can happen. Toxins can store in layers and when one layer is removed, you can uncover another deeper layer that needs to be removed. Just remember that you are getting healthier as you rid the body of dead and toxic debris.

Did you know that all raw foods, including raw meats, eggs and dairy have a negative ionic charge? This is important to understand because toxins have a positive charge. Because opposites attract, the negative charge from raw foods can bind with the positive charge of toxins to eliminate them from the body. It is interesting that all cooked foods have a positive charge (toxins). Therefore, when you ingest foods in their raw form, they assist in the detoxification process due to their negative charge and they serve as nutrients to feed every cell in our body.

Raw Fats
Raw fats are one of the most crucial foods required for radiant health. Yes, I just said fat! Raw fats come in the form of raw eggs, raw unpasteurized dairy (milk, cream, kefir, cheese and butter), raw coconut cream or truly unheated coconut oil, raw avocado and unheated virgin or extra virgin olive oil. Their importance is vital to protect, soften, lubricate, cleanse, rebuild and fuel the body. Repeated studies have shown that diets low in fat have been associated with depression, cancer, psychological disorders, fatigue, suicide and violence. Harvard University proved that the modern day, low fat diet has caused an alarming increase in degenerative disorders. I find it very

interesting that my uncle developed Parkinson's disease, a neurological disorder, less than two years after going on a no fat diet.

Did you know that nearly two thirds of the human brain is fat? Myelin, the protective sheath that covers communication neurons of the brain is 70% fat. We desperately need beneficial raw fats and cholesterol to maintain healthy brain and nervous system function.

Fats should not be feared in their raw form. They lubricate the brain, arteries, the gastrointestinal system and all organs in the body, including the skin. When raw fats are combined with raw meats, they assist the body in cell regeneration.

Raw fats also protect the body from toxins by binding with them so the toxins can be removed safely. Shortly after I had numerous mercury amalgams removed from my mouth, I began experiencing a burning in my esophagus and stomach. It was excruciatingly painful. I realized the toxic mercury was dumping into my GI tract for removal from my body. Because I did not have enough fats in my diet at the time, the mercury was damaging my GI tract on its way out of my body. I immediately started drinking a mixture of raw eggs, raw cream and raw unheated honey. The pain disappeared in 10 minutes. I continued to drink this mixture to coat and protect my esophagus for two weeks. I needed the mucus layer for protection against the toxic metals. The mercury could bind with the fats and protect my organs on its way out of my body. I occasionally experience this same GI pain when I am dumping toxins, and immediately go to a diet almost exclusively of raw cream, raw milk, raw eggs and raw honey. It works for me every time.

Raw diary has been shown to be one of the most beneficial and healing foods around. Raw milk was used by ancient physicians

Hippocrates and Galen to cure diseases, by Dr. J.E. Crewe of the Mayo Foundation to cure TB, high blood pressure, prostate disease, diabetes, kidney disease, chronic fatigue and obesity. Large amounts of raw butter have been successfully used to heal autism in children. The fat in the butter heals and protects the nerve cells (myelin) in the brain and heals leaky gut also found in autistic patients.

Raw dairy products provide an excellent source of raw fat. Nature gives us an abundance of animals that provide health giving milk: cow, sheep, goats, camels, buffalo, yaks, oxen, antelope, reindeer and zebras. The milk can be consumed as is, or made into kefir that is full of good bacteria. The cream from the milk can also be consumed as is or made into butter. Some of the earliest human artifacts include pots that contain traces of milk residue. In fact, historians believe milk consumption dates back at least 30,000 years with the beginning of civilization.

Raw Meats
When it was found that cooking meats causes mutagens that cause cancer, many thought the solution was to not eat meat at all. However, raw meats are crucial to the healing process. They are necessary in regenerating cells in our body. As I described in the section on *detoxification,* after a bacteria, virus, parasite or mold breaks down degenerative tissue for efficient elimination, it is important to our health that we eat the proper foods to then regenerate new cells in this area. This is what raw meat protein does. Raw meats in combination with a raw fat will regenerate new healthy cells faster than any other food. I suggest reading Dr. Vonderplanitz book, *"The Recipe for Living without Disease"* to reference which types of raw meats support regeneration of which specific cells. For example, an excerpt from his book states that, *"White meat such as non-farmed, ocean wild-caught fish and seafood helps reconstitute nerves, including the brain".* No other foods can regenerate

cells as quickly as raw animal protein such as beef, fowl and fish.

Shop around for beef and chicken that is not pumped full of hormones and antibiotics. Grass fed beef (supplemented with organic corn) and free range chicken are the best. A huge amount of soy is being fed to animals these days which is one of the most genetically modified grains out there. Do your best to try to find meats that have not been fed soy. It is highly toxic! It is not easy since it has become a cheap way for farmers to feed their animals. When eating fish, choose wild fish rather than farmed. Again, the feed farmed fish are getting is very poor quality. In fact, in the case of farm raised salmon, they are being given red dye to color the fish. If a farm raised salmon were to not get the red dye in their food, when you cut it open, it would be grey! Many states are now requiring that labeling be put on the farmed salmon stating it has dye in it. Read labels carefully and ask questions.

Raw Vegetables
Drink your vegetables! Because the Standard American Diet is so void of nutrition, this is a great way to pack in the vitamins, minerals, phytonutrients, enzymes and other nutrients we don't even know about. You can throw away your vitamins because fresh raw juice is a perfect nutritional supplement to the rest of your raw diet. Fresh raw green vegetable juices are also important to alkalinize the blood. They help keep us in balance. Another purpose for these juices is to hydrate and oxygenate our cells.

I say green juices because this is what I want you to work toward. Try to limit juices with fruits and root vegetables like carrots and beets because they are high in sugar. I drink celery, cucumber and parsley juice with a little bit of ginger (for taste) every day. It is a good tasting juice, full of essential nutrients.

Try to be conscious of using organic vegetables whenever possible and support your local organic farmer whenever you can. Not only are conventionally raised fruits and vegetables full of pesticides, herbicides and are now irradiated, they are very low in minerals due to the depleted soils they are grown in. A word of caution: Large companies are now starting to jump on the organic "band wagon" and are using their money to lobby Washington to loosen organic standards. Ask your store's produce manager to buy from reputable organic farms.

Raw Fruits

Fruits are also full of high quality nutrients and should be eaten in their raw form. Unlike some raw food eaters, I do not believe they should be eaten in high quantity. It is just too much sugar for most people. When fruits are eaten, it is best to eat a raw fat with them. Avocado, raw cheese, raw eggs and coconut cream with a fruit, or raw cream on berries are all good examples. I like to have my fruit in a smoothie made with raw eggs, coconut cream and raw cream or raw kefir. Raw fruits eaten alone or in quantity can cause extreme mood swings, but the addition of the raw fat helps prevent this from occurring. It is also best to eat fruits in the afternoon so the fruit sugars will not affect mood. However, there are times when I eat smoothies on the run in the morning or give my daughter smoothies for breakfast to get some protein in her. When starting on a raw diet, transition is key and if that works best for you, sometimes you need to do it. I know many people that started eating raw with a morning smoothie and do very well with it, while others need to wait until afternoon to consume their fruit.

Raw Nuts

Raw nuts can be eaten, but be wary that the body cannot digest large amounts of them. Think about how nuts are found in the wild. It takes quite a long time to remove the shell from most nuts to get to the edible center. If we were to eat them in the wild, we would probably eat only small amounts and very slowly. Modern day machinery has made it easy to buy packages of already shelled nuts and thus easy to overeat them. Nuts contain enzyme inhibitors such as phytic acid that prevent proper digestion, can cause mineral loss and can interfere with protein absorption. This is why some cultures have been known to soak or sprout them, to deactivate the enzyme inhibitors. I personally have tried soaked nuts and cannot tolerate them. I think they taste awful! I like to eat them as a "Nut Formula" (as described in the book *"The Recipe for Living Without Disease"*). This combines raw nuts with raw butter, raw eggs and raw honey. This combination neutralizes the enzyme inhibitors and tastes delicious!

Raw Honey
When I refer to raw honey, I am referring to honey that has come right from the hive without any sort of heat application. Raw, unheated honey is in its pure form and has not been subjected to any kind of heat during its processing or packaging. Raw honey is being rediscovered for its medicinal qualities. It has more than 75 different compounds, is loaded with enzymes and is being touted as one of today's "Superfoods". Enzymes are catalysts for biochemical reactions in the body and are necessary for our bodies to function properly. They are found in nearly all raw foods and are high in raw honey. Cooking food kills these necessary enzymes. Raw honey replaces enzymes needed throughout the body. Honey that is heated over 93 degrees F causes damage to natural insulin-like substances in it. When honey is heated over 104 degrees F, it turns into radical sugar that is so toxic that it destroys cellular membranes and acts like regular table sugar in the body.

Raw, unheated honey, in combination with natural mineral water and lemon, has been used for over 5000 years in Ayurvedic medicine for weight loss. Ancient medical scriptures show the benefits of honey include: improved digestion, improved eyesight, soothes a sore throat, gives suppleness to your body, purifies and heals ulcers, gives color to complexion, improves intelligence, cures many types of disease, and heals wounds. In fact, Dr. P.C. Molan published a report summarizing over 97 different studies on the effects of raw honey. His report is entitled, *"Honey as a Dressing for Wounds, Burns and Ulcers: A Brief Review of Clinical Reports and Experimental Studies"*.

The following are just some of results reported:

- Infection is rapidly cleared
- Inflammation and swelling quickly reduced
- Odor is reduced
- Sloughing of necrotic tissue is induced
- Healing occurs rapidly with minimal scarring
- Caused no tissue damage
- Promotes the healing process
- Burns heal rapidly without secondary infection
- Sloughs gangrenous tissue
- Increased blood flow in wounds noticed
- Healed ulcers & burns faster than any other local application used before
- Helps skin regenerate, making plastic reconstructive surgery unnecessary
- Reduces edema
- Reduces pain from burns

Nearly all honey sold in grocery stores and even most of the honey sold in health food stores is heated. Just because a label says "raw honey" does not mean it is really raw. It needs to say, raw, unheated, unprocessed. And then, sometimes they are still not telling the truth. It is suggested that you call the company that packaged the honey to find out what exact temperatures were reached at any time of processing and packaging. Smoking the hives is also heating the honey. I have personally spoken to numerous companies that insist their honey is truly raw and when I question them further, I find out that they actually do heat it to sometimes over 115 degrees F to soften it for packaging. Most raw honeys crystallize very quickly so they can be difficult to use in recipes. The raw, unheated sage honey (available on my website) does not crystallize for a very long time and is easy to use in recipes. It is also packaged in glass jars so there is no leeching of plastic chemicals into the honey from the plastic containers.

Additionally, raw honey works as a preservative in your green juices and was used by indigenous cultures as a preservative in herbal medicines. You can make three days worth of juice by blending a small amount of raw honey in it, pouring the juice into canning jars (such as Ball jars) with very little or no air in it and refrigerating.

Additional Raw Ingredients
There are other raw ingredients that can be used in recipes when preparing foods. These include raw apple cider vinegar, spicy peppers, herbs like fresh basil, mint, rosemary and other ingredients such as raw carob. Dried spices can be used as well, but make sure to use a quality brand of organic spices as most all non-organic dried spices have been irradiated.

Proof/Support for Eating Raw

Dr Weston Price, a dentist from Cleveland, Ohio, noticed that his patients were developing more and more chronic and degenerative diseases than ever and that his young patients were coming in with deformed arches and cavities and crooked teeth. He also noticed a correlation between the number of cavities in a person and disease in the body. Dr. Price was noted for his studies on vibrantly healthy indigenous cultures and their relationship to raw foods. On his travels around the world in the 30's and 40's, he found primitive cultures with superior health and no degenerative diseases such as cancer or heart disease. The diets of these people consisted of raw (sometimes fermented) animal products including raw meats, raw eggs, and raw diary. The bulk of the raw animal products these cultures consumed included organ meats and meat fat. Organ meats have the highest level of nutrients and some cultures actually throw away the muscle meats, which we in our culture normally eat, to eat only the organs.

A physician by the name of Dr. Frances Pottenger was well known for his studies with cats. In one of his studies, he fed half of his sick cats raw milk and raw meats, while the other half of his cats were fed the exact same foods, only the meats were cooked and the milk was pasteurized. The cats that were fed the cooked foods developed our modern day degenerative diseases, while the cats that were fed the raw foods were free of disease generation after generation. Upon autopsy of the cats, the ones on the raw diet had healthy pink organs and strong healthy bones. The cats that ate cooked foods had severe degeneration and deteriorated organs as well as osteoporosis of their bones.

A study by a group of Austrian scientists (and published in the prestigious British journal *The Lancet*) reported the findings of 812 children as they relate to allergies, asthma and skin problems.   319 of the children had grown up with regular exposure to a farm, including drinking of raw unpasteurized "farm milk". The other 493 were non-farm children. The study found that only 1 % of the farm children showed any signs of asthma as compared to 11% of the non-farm children. 3% of the farm children showed signs of hay fever as compared to 13% of the non-farm children.

Jordan Rubin, NMD, CNC, in his book, *"Patient Heal Thyself,"* says, "A lot of diseases, we now realize, result from living too far removed from our microscopic allies, the beneficial bacteria in our environment". He talks about how dirt (or the Earth's soil) when untouched by pesticides, herbicides and other forms or irradiation, is full of beneficial microbes. He goes on to prove how children that are exposed to this soil are healthier than those that are kept away from it. The probiotics found in soil naturally is beneficial for the GI tract. When probiotics are separated from their food source, (a process most supplement manufacturers currently do), the end product needs to be refrigerated in order for that probiotic to remain alive. As soon as you ingest that source into a warm body, is it actually giving you the benefits you desire? When you get your probiotic from a raw food source such as fermented dairy or meats, it is in its complete, whole food form, stable in the body.

Vilhjalmur Stefansson was an anthropologist, an extremely well known explorer and writer. He was educated at University of North Dakota, State University of Iowa and Harvard. During his years living with and studying the Eskimos, he noticed they lived on a diet of about 90% raw meat and fish with virtually zero carbohydrates, and were free of our modern day diseases.

He was so convinced that nutritionists were mistaken to recommend the "balanced diet" that we currently know, that he and a fellow explorer, Karsten Anderson, agreed to a study where they ate only meat and water for one year (two pounds of lean meat to a half pound of fat). After one year, Stefansson who had been eating the way Eskimos ate for years remained in excellent health, while Anderson was in far better physical condition and health than when he started the diet.

Raw Food Combining

Although all raw foods *can* be eaten together, there are certain combinations that work best to not disturb digestion and assimilation of that particular food. It is really very simple:

Raw fats and raw unheated honey can (and usually should) be eaten with any other raw food such as meats, juices, nuts and fruits.

Raw vegetable juices and raw meats should be eaten separately from one another and 45 minutes or more apart. These foods can interfere with the digestion of one another.

Eating these foods separately prevents interference with the digestion or healing effects of that particular food. For example, eating vegetables with meat protein can interfere with the digestion of the protein and cause gas.

If you do eat salads, try to eat them as your last meal of the day. On a raw diet, the roughage from the vegetables takes a long time to break down and move through the system. Allow for at least 4-5 hours for that to happen by eating it as your last meal before bed. This gives it the entire night to digest. If you were to eat raw meat protein (for example) after a salad, the salad would hold up the meat protein from digestion and assimilating properly. Raw foods move in a much different way than cooked food.

Digestion & Elimination

There is no comparison to raw foods when it comes to digestion and elimination. Your body knows exactly what to do with food in its purest raw form. Unlike cooked food that sits in your GI tract, putrefies and makes you feel bloated for hours, raw food is broken down quickly and the nutrients are absorbed into various areas of the body but never leave you with a bloated or stuffed feeling. The body uses nearly all of the raw food with very little left as waste.

Raw foods move through the body much more quickly than cooked foods. Colonics are fast becoming the "in" thing because cooked food putrefies and accumulates in the intestinal tract. On a fully raw diet that has plenty of raw fats, colonics are not needed. The raw fats lubricate the intestinal tract allowing for frequent elimination and the absorption of toxins.

I personally do not believe in colonics. It is not a natural process and removes the important intestinal flora. They can also become addicting, especially when on a cooked diet. One feels bloated and backed up, so they go in for a colonic to move the stored waste from the cooked food. Of course that person feels better, so they go back again and again. Over time, the colon, which is a muscle, could potentially stop working the way it normally should because it counted on the colonic to do the work for it.

Diseases Cured by Raw Foods

Raw foods will change your life! I have seen what eating raw can do to drastically change a person's ill health around. I know what it has done for me personally and I have met numerous people that have reversed "so called" incurable diseases such as cancer, diabetes, chronic fatigue, lymphoma, etc. I highly recommend Dr. Aajonus Vonderplanitz book, "*We Want to Live*". The second half of the book describes nearly every ailment you can think of, what their causes are and specific foods to eat to treat them. This is a must have for anyone who wants to get truly healthy.

The fastest growing alternative practice and a wonderful tool for assessing your health is Iridology. Iridology is the study of the iris to diagnose disease. Every part of the body (including organs, glands and tissues) are represented in the iris and discolorations show disease and weaknesses. An Iridologist uses a special camera to photograph the eye and because of today's technology, it can be viewed immediately on a computer. Because the iris shows what is occurring at the cellular level, it is possible to detect disease that is just beginning in the body, even before our modern day diagnostic tools can detect them or symptoms show.

I have found that Iridologists generally have two thoughts regarding true eye color. Some believe that the eyes of truly healthy individuals are one of two colors: blue or amber while others believe all eyes to be blue. That means that when all of the disease is removed from a body and the flecks and discolorations are gone, one of these two colors will be the "true" color of the eye.

My own eyes started out a brownish, green color with two-thirds of my iris being dark brown. I have seen drastic color changes occur since I have been on a raw diet and the dark brown is fading away to expose more green and even blue is coming through. As I continue on a raw diet, I will some day have blue eyes! I keep the photographs of my irises out on my desk to remind me of how healthy I am getting.

If all disease is a form of toxemia in the body, it is possible to rid the body of these toxins and free yourself of disease. I truly believe it is possible to reverse almost any disease if caught early enough. It took many years to accumulate them and it will take time to eliminate them as well, so be patient and be healthy.

Vitamins & Supplements

We know that vitamins and minerals are crucial to health and in the prevention of disease. I am often asked about vitamins, antioxidants and supplements. Judith DeCava, MS, LCN, CCN, wrote an amazing book on this subject titled *"The Real Truth about Vitamins and Antioxidants"*, and defines a vitamin as, "a group of chemically related compounds". They are very complex mechanisms, woven together, that work synergistically. "A vitamin consists of, not only the organic nutrient(s) identified as the vitamin, but also enzymes, coenzymes, antioxidants, and trace element activators...Enzyme activators may include trace elements such as manganese, cobalt, zinc, copper, selenium, vanadium, and so on. These components are effective only when in the proper organic (organized) state. A vitamin supplement...must contain all the factors indigenous to food that make up the vitamin's organic unity and entirety". Basically, she is stating that a specific vitamin is made up of numerous components and that it only works the way it is designed to work when it is complete. When a vitamin company tries to reproduce that vitamin, it is virtually impossible because of the complex compounds within a specific vitamin that are still unknown. A man-made vitamin is missing components.

Vitamin supplements sold in stores come in various forms and it is very important to understand their differences. There are three basic kinds of vitamins, **fractionated, synthetic** and **whole food** vitamins. When a vitamin is sold in its **fractionated form**, it is not the complex group of compounds found in whole food form.   For example: Vitamin C is a complex compound of over 150 anticarcinogens, redox agents and other phytochemicals.   It is not uncommon to find one single compound like ascorbic acid or citric acid sold as "vitamin C". This is NOT vitamin C. It is one single compound of vitamin C.   Another example is with vitamin E.   Alpha tocopherol is commonly sold as vitamin E.   In fact Vitamin E is a complex compound of several tocopherols and tocotrienols.   Alpha tocopherol is NOT vitamin E.   When a person takes the single fractionated "supplement", he is putting himself in danger. Taking one single compound throws off the balance of the entire complex in the body.   DeCava says, "Taking one or any number of such vitamin parts can create an imbalance of vitamins, which is worse than a deficiency".   Numerous studies have shown that animals fed a diet lacking a certain vitamin did far better than animals given that vitamin in a fractionated form.

Synthetic vitamins are synthesized in a laboratory: in other words, they are chemically made. Although synthetic vitamins may have the exact same chemical characteristics (or molecular formula) as a vitamin in its natural state from a food, the synthetic vitamins contain "mirror images" of some of the compounds. A mirror image of something is the opposite of that thing in its "natural" state.   Therefore, the synthetic vitamins with its "mirror image" compounds are going to do the opposite of what they were intended to do. Dr. Gilbert Levin, says, "...a left-handed molecule cannot take part in chemical reactions meant for a right-handed molecule any more than a left hand can fit in a right-handed glove...its odd geometry (arrangement, configuration) would prevent it from being metabolized (processed) by the body." A doctor from one of the largest pharmaceutical companies in the U.S. called these components "useless" and "often poisonous".

The third kind of supplement is a **whole food** vitamin. Many believe that these are far superior to fractionated or synthetic supplements. Most of them are made by taking an actual food (usually raw), dehydrating or freeze drying it and then grinding it up and putting into capsules. Although this is better than the other forms of vitamins, I cannot believe that putting a real live food through this process can actually preserve all of the vital nutrients. I believe that at least some of them are lost in the process. That brings us back to the problem of putting something that is not in its balanced form into the body. It throws off the synergistic complex. In addition, the body can only utilize approximately 2-12% of these supplements properly which leaves 88-98% as waste. In order to eliminate this waste, the body uses up vital nutrients.

A "live", unadulterated whole food is the only way to get the most complete form of vitamins and minerals. Judith DeCava says, "The point is that whole foods contain all of the related nutrients - vitamins, minerals, trace elements, enzymes, coenzymes, amino acids, fatty acids, etc. - that function together for the biochemical equilibrium of the human body. Supplying single vitamins in supplements, separated fractions or synthetic chemicals can be harmful and lead to further depletions and imbalances".

Enzymes: A Vital Component to Health

Most people know very little about enzymes other than the fact that they are in our food. Leading enzymes specialists believe they are one of the most vital components to health and well being. Dr. Edward Howell, a biochemist and nutritional researcher, was a leader in enzyme research, and has documented over fifty years of research on the effects of enzymes on human health. In his book, *"Enzyme Nutrition: The Food Enzyme Concept"*, he proves that a lack of enzymes in the body "can lead to serious illness and even death".

First, let's talk enzyme basics. There are three different categories of enzymes: *metabolic, digestive* and *food enzymes.* Every organ and tissue in the body depends on **metabolic enzymes** for survival because they are responsible for repairing damage. Each organ and tissue has its own specific set of metabolic enzymes designed to repair that specific organ or tissue. Without these vital metabolic enzymes, organs and tissues could not survive, and eventually the body will not survive.

Digestive enzymes do exactly what the name refers to...they digest the food we eat so the vital nutrients can be assimilated in the body. Where metabolic and digestive enzymes are made within our body, the third category, **food enzymes**, come from the foods we eat. Food enzymes are helpers; they start food digestion so the body doesn't need to produce so many digestive enzymes to digest the food. Food enzymes are highly susceptible to heat and can be damaged at temperatures as low as 96 degrees F. All cooked and processed foods are completely void of food enzymes. They are destroyed to prevent color changes and preserve the food that would naturally be broken down by the enzymes.

We each have a fixed amount of enzymes that can be produced by the body in our lifetime, what Dr. Howell refers to as our "enzyme potential". On a raw food diet, the food enzymes begin digestion of the food we eat; therefore, few digestive enzymes are needed, leaving ample metabolic enzymes for running the body. When we eat cooked food, our bodies manufacture some of these digestive enzymes to digest food, but because the cooked food is completely void of food enzymes that would have assisted in the digestion process, the pancreas and other digestive organs are forced to secrete large amounts of digestive enzymes, causing great stress on these organs and limiting the amount of metabolic enzymes that can be produced to heal, repair and run our organs and tissues. If our organs are not being healed and repaired, numerous health problems could occur. On a cooked diet, it is not uncommon to see a weakened and/or enlarged pancreas due to it being overworked.

You can see how day after day, and year after year, vital enzymes are being wasted due to all of the cooked and processed foods we ingest. When we are young, we have the large pool of "enzyme potential" to draw from, but as we age and our pool is depleted, eating cooked foods becomes more stressful on the body. A lack of metabolic enzymes in a particular organ or tissue can lead to weakness, disease and even death. Everyone on a standard American diet has disease in the body. It is not always noticeable until later in life (although it seems debilitating diseases are being diagnosed at younger and younger ages), but it is there.

Raw nuts, seeds and grains (such as raw wheat germ) contain enzyme inhibitors. When these foods are eaten, the inhibitors cause a great outpouring (or wasting) of digestive enzymes, again leaving fewer metabolic enzymes to do their work. Dr. Howell talks of an experiment where "young rats and chickens were fed a diet of raw soybeans (high in enzyme inhibitors) and huge quantities of pancreatic digestive enzymes were wasted in combating the inhibitors. The pancreas gland enlarged to handle the extra burden, and the animals sickened and failed to grow".

Eating Out

Most of us eat out to socialize. It is a bonus to have good food. We live in a culture of such isolation, each of us live in our own little apartment or house, we work in a cubicle, office or out of our car. We have a human need to be social with other people (our friends, family or coworkers). It is an important thing. I like to eat out even if I am alone just to have the energy of other people around me. I don't even have to know anyone! Eating raw does not prevent you from having your nights out to dinner.

It is not that difficult to eat out when on a raw diet. I eat out three or four nights a week. Here is all you need to know. First of all, Sushi has never been hotter than right now and nearly everyone has at least one good Sushi restaurant they could frequent. My seven-year-old daughter and I can eat an impressive amount of sushi. Also, I am pleasantly surprised as to how many restaurants are offering *Ceviche, Tartare* and *Carpaccio* (all raw meats) these days. *Ceviche* is usually sold at Mexican restaurants (but available at other kinds of restaurants as well). It is made with raw fish marinated in a lemon or lime juice with various vegetables and spices. *Tartare* can be made with either fish or red meat, and *Carpaccio* is usually made with some sort of red meat. I live in a very small town and I can think of at least 10 different restaurants that offer raw meats. Most of them are offered as appetizers, so I order a double appetizer brought out on one plate when everyone else gets their main course. Start checking menus. If your favorite restaurant does not offer a *Ceviche, Tartar* or *Carpaccio,* ask them to start making one. Tell them how popular and healthy raw foods are and how you will frequent their business more if they were to offer at least one. It is amazing what will happen once customers start demanding that more raw foods be served. Your voice will make a difference.

When I am going out to a place that I know does not have any sort of raw meat on their menu, or if I am really hungry and know that I will not be filled up by what raw meats a restaurant will offer me, I eat my meat meal first, before I leave the house. Then, I can either get a raw meat appetizer to supplement what I have eaten before I left the house, or get a big salad if it is dinner time, since it will be the last meal of the day and that will allow enough time for the roughage to digest before my next meal in the morning.

Once you start eating raw, you will be so amazed at how you feel when you leave the restaurant as compared to the others in your party that just ate a cooked meal. Listen to them...."I am so full", "Does anyone have any antacids?", "I am stuffed", "I don't feel good", "I have to get to sleep". You will never feel this way on a raw diet. You will always be satisfied without that overstuffed feeling. Note: Over time as your body rids itself of toxins, you may notice a slight headache or stomach ache from eating raw meats in restaurants. This happens due to the amount of sodium they use in sauces they put on their meats. You may need to start asking them to bring the dishes with sauces on the side or without the sauces at all. Chefs are so used to needing salt to flavor cooked meats that they put it in raw meat dishes as well. You will see that meats in their raw form are full of flavor and most do not need sauces, especially salt.

People often ask me what I do for "fast food". "What if you are out running errands and the time flies by and you need a quick snack?" You have a few choices. Try to plan for this by taking the food you will need for the next few hours with you.

Sometimes if I am famished and need some serious food immediately, I will stop by a market and pick up a hormone and antibiotic free filet steak. I usually sit in my car or at one of the tables at the store and cut it up with a plastic knife and eat it (either alone or with some fresh store-made guacamole) Or, sometimes you can find a good market that has a quality pre-made sushi. This is a favorite with raw beginners.

Weight

Doctors have been telling us that weight is a determinant of heart disease and many other diseases. That is true on a cooked diet. It is not true on a raw diet. The reason it holds true for a cooked diet is because the cooked foods produce toxins that store in the body, producing toxemia that can cause various conditions. Cooked fats and cholesterol accumulate over time causing hardened arteries, nerve endings, lymph nodes, etc. It is then obvious that the heavier a person is, the more stored toxins and toxic fats they have in their body. Most obese people eat huge amounts of processed foods, including cooked vegetable oils. Nearly all processed foods contain these oils. Read labels and you will see.

Likewise, being thin does not necessarily mean you are healthy if on a cooked diet. In fact, a thin person can sometimes be at a greater risk because they have no fat reserves on their body to protect them from toxins. Toxins will store in fat first before organs. A thin person has no protection from our toxic environment or the byproducts produced from cooking foods. A thin person needs to be sure they are getting enough raw fats in their diet every day.

Toxins embedded deep into cells need to be removed through a weight gain and loss process. Because toxins store in fat, the only way to get to these deeply embedded toxins are to put extra weight on the body with raw fats. These raw fats store in the cells, the toxins store in the fat and then the fat is lost (eliminated) along with the toxins.

Without even trying, my own body regularly goes through a cycle of weight gain and loss on its own. My weight goes up and down 5-8 lbs throughout the year. Nature automatically does what it needs for me.

Something else that needs to be addressed regarding weight is the following: We know that as we age our organs shrink and degenerate. Look at the obvious organ, our skin. It dries out and shrivels up. Degenerative organs weigh less than healthy organs because degenerative tissue is less dense. Healthy organs are denser and weigh more. As every organ (e.g. liver, spleen, heart, lungs, pancreas, kidneys, gallbladder, muscles, ligaments, tendons and the list goes on) gets healthier (denser) you may begin to weigh more. I found myself gaining weight but my clothes still fit the same. In other words, rejoice! Do not pay attention to the scale, it means nothing at this point. Again, it is the idea that my organs have gotten denser, thus they weigh more. On a raw foods diet, underweight people will gain weight and overweight people will lose weight as our bodies balance itself out.

Water

On a raw diet you will not need to drink as much water as someone eating cooked foods. This is because all raw foods have water in them and you are taking in large amounts of water throughout the day in the foods you eat. A person on a cooked food diet needs the additional water intake because the cooking and dehydrating of food removes the water content. When that person eats the cooked foods, water is pulled from their body to re-hydrate the foods, thus leeching water from the body. All raw foods, such as raw eggs, raw meats, fresh raw juices, raw fruits and vegetables and smoothies, contain water. I only drink about 8 to 16 ounces of water each day (depending on my physical exertion that day) and I never drink water with a meal. Drinking any kind of liquid with a meal dilutes stomach acids that are necessary to breakdown our foods. This can interfere with digestion and absorption of the foods and nutrients into our system.

Naturally sparkling mineral water is a good, relatively clean, source of water to drink and most of these waters come in glass bottles, which I prefer. Plastic bottles leech toxins into the water. Make sure it says "naturally sparkling mineral water", not "sparkling natural mineral water". The latter means they have taken mineral water and added CO_2 to make it sparkling. Naturally sparkling mineral water with raw honey mixed in is a good remedy for a toxic blood headache and constipation.

Bottled *spring water* comes from a natural spring and contains all of its natural minerals. Nothing has been removed or added.

This too is ok to drink, but is almost always bottled in plastic. Also, check the source by calling the company or on the internet. Some spring waters are from protected pristine springs and some are from a local spring that may have come in contact with agricultural pollutants.

Tap water can come from either a public water system or a well. If it is from a *public water* system, it has been treated with large amounts of chemicals such as fluoride, chlorine and chloramines. When chlorine in public water mixes with organic matter already in the water, chloroform is formed. Chloroform has been proven to cause damage to the central nervous system, liver and kidneys and is thought to be a carcinogen. Read more about this in *Home Safe Home*, by Debra Lynn Dadd. *Well water* comes from an aquifer deep below the ground that has been tapped. This water also contains the natural minerals from the earth, but should always be tested for chemicals before consumption. Sometimes agricultural chemicals such as pesticides and herbicides (more carcinogens) get into this water and poison it. Well water sometimes has a strong sulfur smell and is difficult to drink by most people.

Many people these days are purifying their water. I live in an area that has city water loaded with toxic chemicals. I have a "whole house" purifier to remove these chemicals from our bath and shower. Debra Lynn Dodd writes, "According to a study done by the Massachussetts Department of Environmental Quality Engineering published in the *American Journal of Public Health*, 29 to 46 percent of water pollutant exposure (depending on the chemical and the concentration) occurs through the skin in children, and 50 to 70 percent in adults!" The skin is the largest organ and "with skin absorption, virtually 100 percent of the contaminants go directly into the bloodstream." Along with my whole house purifier, I also have a reverse osmosis purifier for our drinking water. It removes virtually all contaminants. Unfortunately, it also removes minerals as well. To replace these minerals, I add *Terramin* clay to my water (available on my website www.RawToRadiant.com). This specific type of living clay has the perfect proportion of minerals in it as well as the smallest particle size to guarantee absorption into the cells. Read more about this in section two.

When you take a shower or bath, the chemicals in the water are heated and turn into a vapor. Vapors are then breathed in and are said to be even more toxic than the liquid form of the chemical.

Following are just some of the chemicals found in tap water:
- Chlorine
- Chloramine
- Fluoride
- Nitrates
- Pesticides
- Herbicides
- Industrial solvents

Pipes can leech:
- Cadmium
- Lead
- Asbestos

Polyvinyl Chloride (PVC) pipes can leech:
- Methyl Ethyl Ketone (MEK)
- Dimethyl-form amide (DMF)
- Cyclohexanone (CH)
- Tetrahydrofuran (THF)
- Carbon tetrachloride
- Tetrachloroethene
- Trichloroethane
- Dibutyl phthalate
- Vinyl Chloride

These are known carcinogens that cause birth defects, cancer, heart disease, neurological system problems, headaches and probably a whole list of issues we don't even know about yet. There is a commercial I remember that used to run showing a pregnant mother, standing at the sink in her kitchen, drinking a glass of tap water. The voice over says, "a little lead won't hurt me." Then they showed her drinking it over and over and over and over... It is not the one swallow that will hurt anyone; it is the accumulation of toxins from various sources throughout the years over and over that will literally destroy us. That is why it is so important to detoxify on an ongoing basis and rebuild our bodies through raw foods.

Distilled water is another form of purified water. Long term use of distilled water can literally kill you. It has been stripped completely of everything in it, is highly acidic and will cause every part of your body to leech nutrients, especially electrolytes such as sodium, potassium and chloride as well as trace minerals like magnesium. Paavo Airola was known for writing about the dangers of drinking distilled water in the 1970's, and more recently Zolton P. Rona, M.D. wrote an article titled, *"Early Death Comes from Drinking Distilled Water."*

Lifestyle Changes

As you start your journey of incorporating more raw foods into your life and you begin detoxifying your body, you will start feeling better. The cleaner you get, the better you will feel over time. As this process unfolds, you may become aware of the products you are using on a daily basis and the chemicals/toxins they have in them. Our skin is the largest organ of our body. Everything we put on our skin will absorb right into it. Since we are trying to detoxify our bodies, we don't want to put chemicals back into it if we can help it. We are bombarded with toxins everyday that we have no control over. So, if we have an opportunity to take control of some things, we need to do so.

Start watching for the following ingredients in shampoos, skin care products, deodorants and cosmetics:

- Sodium laurel sulfate
- Parabens (anything ending in ...paraben)
- Ethylenediaminetetraacetic acid (EDTA)
- Selenium Sulfide
- Fluoride
- Aluminum
- Chlorine
- Alcohol
- Mineral Oil
- Talc
- Ammonia
- Formaldehyde

- Triclosan
- BNPD
- TEA
- DEA

Nearly all of the ingredients on labels that we cannot pronounce are toxic chemicals. *Formaldehyde* is often used as a preservative and hidden under the name quaternium-15. I urge you to read the book *"Home Safe Home"*. In it, Deborah Lynn Dadd tells you exactly what is in all of the products in your home, such as *selenium sulfide* in dandruff shampoos, which if swallowed, cause vital organ degeneration.

Parabens have been found in the breast tissue of women with breast cancer and are another chemical that is found in nearly every line of skin care, shampoos & conditioners and deodorants. Parabens are used as a preservative and can absorb into the skin after being applied. Some are easy to spot on labels because they use "paraben" in their name such as: benzylparaben, isobutylparaben, butylparaben, ethylparaben and n-propylparaben. However, the chemical industry is aware that consumers are becoming educated and are now using all kinds of different names for parabens such as benzoic acid, 4-hydroxy-, 2-methylpropyl ester, aseptoform butyl and the list goes on and on and on. Go to my website for a link to a page with all of the different names parabens are being sold under.

Start looking for healthier alternatives for:

Toothpaste
Soap
Deodorant
Laundry detergent
Fabric Softener
Household cleaning supplies
Shampoos
Conditioners
Moisturizers

Cosmetics

All natural food stores carry various products, but beware -- just because it is sold in a natural food store does not mean it is necessarily healthy. Read the labels carefully.

Change is a gradual process for most. Start with fluoride-free toothpaste and then switch to aluminum free deodorant and so on. Just do what makes you feel comfortable, and when you are ready to take another step, you will. Over the years, I have been able to change everything to a natural alternative except for one. I have colored or highlighted my hair for years and that has always been the one thing I could not give up. I am finally experimenting with alternatives such as natural hennas (a powder made from plant sources) and herbs. My point is that you don't have to change everything at once and immediately. Be patient with yourself and know that every little change is beneficial.

Equipment

JUICERS:
I highly recommend the Green Star juicer which is a twin gear and works like a press as opposed to a disc spinning juicer (centrifugal ejection). Because the Green Star juicer presses the juice out, it produces juices with:

- The lowest temperature
- The slowest oxidation and fermentation process
- The lowest DNA, enzymatic and mineral degeneration
- The most overall stability
- The highest mineral content
- The highest alkalinity
- The most enhanced bioavailability
- The greatest concentration of oxygen

When using a centrifugal ejection juicer, you can loose a large amount of nutrients due to the oxidation process and due to the heat that can be generated from them. The Green Star is a bit more expensive, but does the best job and is incredibly durable. In fact, it is the only juicer I know that can juice the flesh of a coconut to make coconut cream.

If the Green Star is too pricey for you, shop around and get what you can afford at this time. It is important to get your juice in any way you can.

CITRUS JUICER:
Although it is possible to juice citrus in the Green Star, it is quicker to use an actual citrus juicer. When I make Ceviche', for example, I use limes to marinate the fish. If I were to put the limes through the Green Star with the peel on, the juice would be way too tart; so the limes need to be peeled first, which is too time consuming. An actual citrus juicer works best. I have tried them all and there are two that I highly recommend. The first is an old-fashioned glass juicer that you press the citrus down onto to extract the juice. The second is a stainless steel juicer that you pull a lever down which presses the juice out.

TRAVEL BLENDER/JUICER:
This is a must for all travelers! This blender/juicer combo is perfect for the raw food traveler. Make smoothies and juices right in your hotel room. It is small enough to pack into your suitcase. No more searching for a local juice bar during your travels. These travel blenders/juicers can be bought under the names of Amazing Bullet or Magic Bullet. Shop around for the best price on this.

ICE CREAM MAKER:
Make delicious "raw" home-made ice-cream in 10 minutes with the Donvier ice cream maker. I highly recommend this old fashioned, hand crank maker as it will not emit the electromagnetic radiation of a motorized maker. Once you make your own "healthy" home-made ice cream, you will never want the store bought again. My daughter and I make our own ice cream several times a week.

BLENDERS:
A blender is something you cannot do without and there are three options when it comes to purchasing blenders:

1. A high quality, powerful, industrial type blender is an excellent investment. I recommend either the Total Blender by Blendtech or the Vitamix. Neither are inexpensive, but this is one thing I would invest in. I have tried both and would recommend either one.

2. A simple blender (such as an Oster) where the blade unscrews from the bottom of the blender jar. Blades that detach from blender jars will fit onto any size regular mouth canning jar such as Ball or Kerr. This allows you to use the appropriate size jar for the food you are preparing. For example, I use a quart size jar to make my smoothie every day. I just put my eggs, fruit, honey and cow's cream or coconut cream into the jar, screw on the blade/lid, place it on the blender and turn it on. I take the lid off and drink it right out of the jar. I use small 4 oz. jars to chop nuts or blend honey into my juice to preserve it (see recipes). The canning jars are made of glass, so you don't have to worry about plastic chemicals leaching. This is a must have.

3. You can have both types...I do. I like to use the industrial size when making some foods, and have the option of using the other one when I don't want too much air to get into my foods which will cause oxidation, or if I don't want to blend my foods in plastic.

CANNING JARS:
Canning jars are necessary for use on the regular blenders as listed above. They come in all sizes ranging from 4 oz. to half gallon. I love these because they not only work for blending but because they are air tight and are great for storage as well. I use them for storing all my raw dairy (milk, cream, kefir, etc) and meats. I have donated all of my plastic storage containers and have switched over to glass. It is the safest. Use the tiny 4 ounce jars for snacks in a lunch box in place of plastic.

ANCILLARY ITEMS:
1. Strainer – for straining pulp from juice or for straining coconut water, etc.
2. Knife Set – a good sharp knife set is important.
3. Oyster Shucker – Removes the meat of the coconut to make coconut cream.
4. Cheese Cutter
5. Cutting Board

Visit my website at: www.RawToRadiant.com for most of these products. I have tried to make it a "one stop shop" for people to get these items at a reasonable price.

Section II

Raw Integration

Change is not easy and we all have powerful food addictions that we face each day. I truly believe that food is the number one addiction in this country. Try eliminating your morning cappuccino and see what other food replaces that addiction (if you can even do it). When you have been eating certain foods for 30, 40 or 50+ years, change takes time. Unlike cigarettes or alcohol, we cannot just stop eating. Similarly, most of us cannot just switch over to a 100% raw diet unless faced with a devastating diagnosis such as cancer. There is a realistic way of integrating raw foods into your diet. It is not as hard as you might think it would be as you will be eating most of the same foods as before, just in their raw life giving form.

10 EASY STEPS TO INTEGRATE RAW FOODS INTO YOUR CURRENT DIET

Step 1 - Drink Your Vegetables

Don't change anything you are currently eating. However, I do want you to add one thing...one GREEN juice a day. This is the first step. Our bodies are so acidic from all of the carbohydrates, sugars and cooked proteins we ingest, as well as our blood being acidic from toxins trying to escape, that we need to balance it out. Nearly all fruits and vegetables are alkaline and will contribute to the acid/alkaline balance. However, fruits and root vegetables such as carrots and beets have a lot of sugar and should not been consumed too frequently, especially people with sugar issues.

Because we are so void of nutrients, huge amounts of vegetables and some fruits are necessary every day, to not only meet the daily requirements, but to make up for the missing nutrients in every cell of our body. The most efficient way to assimilate these nutrients into our system is to "Drink our Vegetables". You can get a significant amount of vegetables into one glass of juice. The juice can absorb directly into our system and go immediately to work, without the body having to process all of that roughage. On a totally raw diet, where enough raw fat is ingested, roughage is not necessary. It is only necessary on a cooked diet to push the cooked and processed foods through the intestinal tract. That is because cooked foods do not digest efficiently and they sit in the GI tract left to putrefy and toxins reabsorb into the system.

If you need to start off with a carrot, celery, parsley juice for example, go ahead and do so, but work your way to a totally green juice. I suggest celery, cucumber, parsley and a small amount of ginger (for taste) as a first green drink. I also suggest having the juice strained, if possible. This takes any chunks out of the juice and makes it more palatable.

Step one, as I said, is to drink one 8-12 ounce glass of green juice a day. When you are ready, add a second glass, then a third. Your goal is to drink between 16-32 ounces a day. Really try to get this in your diet. A good way to achieve this is to drink one 12 ounce juice first thing in the morning and your second 12 ounce juice right before bed. If you prefer three 8 ounce juices, drink them first thing in the morning, right before bed and add an additional juice an hour after lunch or an hour before dinner. You'll not believe the difference you will feel when your system reaches an acid/alkaline balance, is receiving huge amounts of nutrients and is being oxygenated.

I am frequently asked about the popular bottled juices found in the stores today. First of all, the majority of them are mostly fruit juice. Labels list ingredients in order of quantity. The first ingredient is what there is most of and the second ingredient is what there is second most of, etc. In nearly all of these juices, the first several ingredients are fruits. That is a significant amount of sugar. The goal is to get green vegetable juices in your system. The second issue I have with them is that they are pasteurized. As I said before, the pasteurization process is at a very high temperature and is designed to kill. It also kills the vital nutrients you are trying to get into your diet. In my opinion, they are not healthy drinks. As far as the green powders are concerned, some are made from whole food vegetables which are on the right track and some are not. However, based on what a vegetable has to go through to get from a fresh wholesome vegetable to a dried out powder, you cannot tell me that nutrients are not lost in that process.

There are a couple of options for getting your daily juice. One is to find a local health food store that makes fresh raw vegetable juices on the spot. If you can stop by and pick one up every day, do so. If not, have them make up two days worth. Drink one and pour the other one into a canning jar (like a Ball jar) to save for the next day. These types of jars can be found in any grocery store and will keep the juice from oxidizing too quickly. Fill the jar to the top so oxygen cannot get in. The second way of getting your juice is to make your own. You can make up to three days worth of juice and preserve it with a little raw honey. See recipes. I highly recommend the Green Star juicer which is a twin gear and works like a press as opposed to a disc spinning juicer (centrifugal ejection).

Step 2 - Eat Meats Raw

If you already like your meats served rare or "black & blue", you are almost there. For the rest of you, start cooking your meats less and less. If you normally cook them well done, gradually transition to medium well, medium, medium rare, rare, black & blue and then finally to raw. Raw meats have great flavor. Many of you may have lost some of your taste bud sensitivity due to all of the salt and seasonings that are needed on cooked foods. Try the recipes in the back of this book for meals like Wild Salmon Ceviche' with avocado, tomato and cilantro or the Buffalo Tartar. I also highly recommend "*Recipes for Living without Disease*", by Aajonus Vonderplanitz. He has created some delicious sauces for various meats!

When I must cook chicken for my daughter, I cook it in water on a gas stove where I can control the heat. I keep the heat (therefore the temperatures) very low until it is done. One other way to cook meats at low temperatures is to use a solar oven. The oven uses the sun to heat up and you can control the temperatures by opening the door. The thermostat registers the lowest temperatures that I have ever seen, below 100 degrees F. Solar ovens can be purchased at www.gaiam.com.

Step 3 - Eat More Sushi

Sushi is hot right now! Everyone is jumping on the Sushi train and for good reason. Raw fish has so many wonderful benefits. It is an animal protein which assists in regeneration of new healthy cells in the body and it is a great source of essential omega-3 fatty acids which have a huge list of benefits including: stabilizing irregular heart beats, reducing blood pressure, protecting against heart and vessel disease, lowering cholesterol and triglyceride levels, is a natural blood thinner which reduces stickiness of blood cells, improves rheumatoid arthritis, improves lupus, improves other autoimmune diseases, improves depression and mental health problems, aids in cancer prevention and the list goes on. The Inuit (Eskimo) people of

Greenland were some of the healthiest humans alive in the 1970's and their diet consisted of very high fats from eating whale, seal and salmon.

I am often asked about the mercury levels in fish from people concerned about heavy metal toxicity. Aajonus Vonderplanitz conducted a study on this very subject. He used swordfish which is known as having one of the highest mercury levels. He measured the level of mercury in the fish before ingesting it (raw) and measured the output of mercury in the urine after eating the fish. 98% of the mercury was excreted into the urine and he believes that the other 2% came out of the body through perspiration. It is his belief that consuming the fish raw is not an issue. It is when the fish is cooked that the mercury becomes a problem. Cooking the mercury changes its chemistry and makes it toxic in humans. I believe the natural raw fat in the fish protects us from much of the toxins and allows us to be able to excrete it from our bodies safely. Heating the fish damages the protective fat and allows for damage from the mercury as well.

I admit I am a sushi junkie! My daughter and I eat sushi three to four nights a week. I eat only sashimi (raw fish only with no rice) but it wasn't always so. I needed to develop a taste for it and I started with rolls and nigiri (fish on top of rice). My daughter on the other hand started eating sashimi when she began eating solids and hasn't stopped since.

I suggest experimenting with different kinds of fish. The wonderful thing about eating fish, especially when it is raw, is that every fish tastes so different. Flavors even vary from different cuts of the fish. For example, the belly of the fish is fatty and has a kind of "melt in your mouth" sensation. Once again, your goal is to eat raw fish with no rice and ask for some sliced avocado on the side (for additional good fat).

Once again, make a transition depending on where you are. If you are a true beginner, start at the top of my sushi order (see below) and if you are experienced, go right for the sashimi. If you need a bit of soy sauce, use it. Eventually you will gain an appreciation of the flavors of each kind of fish and will not need it at all. Some restaurants put different kind of sauces on different kinds of fish as well. Experiment with this and see if you can begin to order them without sauce or with a side of lemon juice for dipping.

Following are some samples of what to order. I have listed them in a progressive order, from what to start out with if you are a beginner, and what to gradually work towards. I have used tuna and salmon as an example, but you can try rolls, nigiri or sashimi with various types of fish.

Cut roll with tuna / avocado/ shiso leaf
Cut roll with wild salmon / avocado/ scallions

Hand roll with very little rice, tuna / avocado/ shiso leaf
Hand roll with very little rice, wild salmon / avocado / scallions

Hand roll with NO RICE: same fish as above.

Nigiri (fish on top of rice): tuna, wild salmon, halibut, sweet shrimp, yellowtail, Aji

Sashimi: raw fish only. I order a wild sashimi platter (nothing cooked). The sushi chefs give me all of the wild fish they have that day.

Try these different types of fish. They all have very different flavors:
* denotes exceptionally good flavor
+denotes a good fish to try as a beginner

Tuna +

Blue fin tuna *+
Yellow fin tuna +
Toro (fatty/belly tuna) *+
Wild Salmon +
Yellow Tail +
Belly cut has more flavor and is fatty *
Spanish Mackerel *+
Stripped Bass +
Halibut +
Rainbow Trout +
Sea Bass +
Swordfish
Oysters - Kumomoto
* Oysters are the best- small little delicacies
Sweet Shrimp
* this is raw, not cooked shrimp
Giant Clam *

A few sushi notes:
Since I have been eating raw and my body is getting so clean, I have not been able to eat soy sauce any more. It gives me a headache. I do eat a bit of "fresh" wasabi with it; or sometimes when I can find my own horseradish root, I will make my own and take it with me to the restaurant. Wasabi has green and blue dye in it, even the so called "fresh" wasabi used by restaurants. There is a brand called *Eden* that is sold in health food stores without dye.

The ginger that is really a bright, pinkish-orange has red dye in it as well; while the natural looking ginger does not, but usually has some sort of sweetener in it.

I used to eat a lot of flying fish eggs and smelt eggs until I found out there is corn syrup mixed in with them. I was told that by a sushi chef from one of the highest quality sushi restaurants. It is mixed in with all of the eggs to keep them fresh so they won't stick together. It is not in quail eggs, since they are broken open right there on the spot. It is only put in caviar eggs like smelt, flying fish, and salmon.

Sushi rice is made with refined sugar and rice vinegar. This is good information to know, so that this knowledge can help support your transition off of sushi rice. Also, grocery and health food stores that sell sushi sometimes put corn syrup in their rice.

Check ingredient labels. Don't assume that just because it is sold in a "health food store", it is healthy. Some grocery stores do not list what is in their rice at all. It just says: "rice". You may have to ask questions.

You can actually make your own sushi at home using raw apple cider vinegar and raw honey to sweeten the rice. Pick up some fresh fish at your local fish market. Kids love to do this!

Step 4 - Cut Out Refined Sugars

Refined, or processed, sugar is one of the most toxic substances we are ingesting. Dr. William Coda Martin was one of the leaders in researching sugar and its toxic effects on the body in the 1950's. When asked "When is food a food and when is it a poison?" He replied that a poison is "Medically: Any substance applied to the body, ingested or developed within the body, which causes or may cause a disease. Physically: Any substance which inhibits the activity of a catalyst which is a minor substance, chemical or enzyme that activates a reaction." Basically, a poison exerts harmful influence. Dr. Martin calls refined sugar "a poison...that is lethal when ingested by humans."

Refined sugar is nothing more than a pure, refined carbohydrate. It is completely void of any vitamins or minerals. Our bodies always want to be in a balanced state, so when a person ingests sugar, our bodies leech vitamins and minerals such as sodium, potassium, magnesium and calcium that the sugar is void of, to achieve that balance. You can see how, as I described in the chapter on vitamins, when we ingest something that is in a fractionated form and not a whole complete state (like a whole raw food), we leech out of our bones, tissues and cells what is needed to make that form complete. Dr. Martin says, "Sugar taken every day produces a continuously over acidic condition, and more and more minerals are required from deep in the body in the attempt to rectify the imbalance. Finally, to protect the blood, so much calcium is taken from the bones and teeth that decay and general weakening begin. Excess sugar eventually affects every organ in the body".

Dr. Joseph Mercola published a list of *"76 Ways Sugar Can Ruin Your Health"* on his website www.mercola.com. The following are some of the reasons from his list:

- Sugar can suppress your immune system
- Sugar can upset mineral relationships in your body
- Sugar can cause high adrenaline and hyperactivity
- Sugar can cause loss of tissue elasticity
- Sugar feeds cancer cells
- Sugar can weaken eyesight
- Sugar can cause premature aging
- Sugar can lead to alcoholism
- Sugar can cause obesity
- Sugar can cause gallstones
- Sugar can cause appendicitis
- Sugar can cause hemorrhoids
- Sugar can cause varicose veins
- Sugar can contribute to osteoporosis
- Sugar can lower vitamin E levels
- Sugar can cause food allergies
- Sugar can impair the structure of your DNA
- Sugar can cause atherosclerosis and cardiovascular disease
- Sugar can cause emphysema

- Sugar intake is higher in people with Parkinson's disease
- Sugar damage pancreas
- Sugar can make tendons more brittle
- Sugar can cause gout
- Sugar can increase your risk of Alzheimer's disease
- Sugar can cause hormonal imbalances
- Sugar increases your risk of Polio

Refined sugars are toxic! Be conscious of what your intake is and what you are giving your family. After you have heightened your awareness of the quantity of sugar you and your family ingest, you can begin to cut back. Especially with kids, make it a slow transition. If sweets are craved, satisfy the craving with fruits or raw unheated honey. For the health of your children, the sooner you stop a sugar addiction the better.

Note: Heated honey, maple syrup, brown sugar and most all forms of sweeteners are no better than your everyday table sugar. The only thing I use in my home is truly raw, unheated, un-smoked honey.

Step 5 - Add Terramin Clay

Terramin clay is a calcium montmorillonite living clay full of macro, micro and trace minerals. Unlike many other types of clay, it has a particle size that is small enough to allow it to pass through cells to get the nutrients inside. It is one thing to ingest clay that has a high amount of nutrients in it, but *Terramin* clay can also get those nutrients inside the cells to nourish them. We know that vitamins will not function properly without trace elements and that enzymes are activated by trace elements, so it is crucial to get them in our diets. Because modern day farming has significantly depleted much of the trace elements from our soil, it is important to supplement our diets with them. Modern day diets that are so void of minerals need the added support of *Terramin* clay.

Terramin clay also has a negative ionic charge that supports the removal of toxins in the body by bonding with the positively charged toxins, allowing them to be eliminated efficiently.

Studies at Cal Tech University show that *Terramin* clay has the three perfect components that allow it to be easily absorbed into the cells which are: It has a particle size of 10-20 microns (smallest available), it has an open negative ionic state, and it has the perfect ratio of minerals.

Terramin clay has no taste and is perfect to put into your drinking water especially if you are drinking purified water that has had the minerals removed through a purification process such as reverse osmosis. You can also put it in juice or smoothies, and it is especially supportive when used in a drink that contains non-organic fruits or vegetables. It will bind with toxins (such as the pesticides and herbicides of non-organic juice) and will allow for the elimination of these toxins.

I highly recommend using *Terramin* clay daily to support alkalinity, the removal of toxins and getting crucial minerals into cells of the body.

Step 6 - Eliminate Processed Foods
As talked about before, processed foods are dead. There is nothing in them to sustain a living human being. In fact, they produce and store even more toxic substances in the body. This usually takes time and you may need to find some transition foods. Start by looking for foods that do not contain cooked vegetable oils. For example, *Newman's Organics* makes one particular kind of pretzel, called *Bavarian Pretzels*, which have no cooked vegetable oils. At my daughter's school, the hottest commodity is seaweed...plain seaweed that has been dried and is used for sushi making. She loves to wrap seaweed around avocado pieces and eat it.

Step 7 - Drink Lemon/Cider Honey Tea

I love this tea. It can be made cold or room temperature by combining naturally sparkling mineral water with raw apple cider vinegar, the juice of a lemon and raw unheated honey. If you prefer a warm drink, warm up some water to a temperature that will not burn your ingredients. Then, add your raw apple cider vinegar, lemon juice and raw honey...so delicious. It will alkalinize your system, and satisfy a sweet tooth. This is also a great transition drink to wean yourself off of coffee.

Step 8 - Add Raw Fats

As I spoke about before, raw fats are crucial in your health. Raw fats include: Raw, unpasteurized dairy (including milk, cream, cheese, butter, kefir, or yogurt), raw unheated coconut oil, coconut cream, raw avocados, raw eggs and unheated virgin or extra virgin olive oil. Start by adding avocados. Eat them with your meat meals, with fruits or just by themselves. Add olive oil by making a salad dressing of olive oil and raw apple cider vinegar for the times you eat salads. Go online to search for raw milk in your area. Once you get it, it won't be hard to get the fat into your diet. Raw unpasteurized milk is so delicious! The taste is far superior to pasteurized milk you buy in the store. Start making home-made ice cream. You won't want store bought again. My favorite home-made ice creams are coconut and pineapple. Yum! We make it almost every night.

Step 9 - Smoothies

Trust me on this one. This is the best smoothie you will ever taste and it has no processed protein powder in it. You will be getting one of the best proteins you can get with the eggs.

Put the following in a blender:

3 raw eggs
1/8 - ¼ of an Organic Pineapple
1 heaping Tablespoon Raw, Unheated Honey

1Tablespoon Coconut Cream or Coconut Oil
1 Tablespoon Raw Cow's Cream (optional)

Blend until mixed well.

Add:

½ bag frozen Organic Strawberries

Blend until strawberries mixed well and it has a thick, frothy consistency.

*Even though I do not advocate frozen foods, it is hard to get fresh berries when they are not in season. If you can get fresh berries, use them instead and put ice cubes in to thicken. The frozen berries or ice cubes are what gives it that frothy consistency and makes it seem like you are eating a desert.

Step 10 - Healthy Snacks
Everyone wants snacks. I suggest starting with transition snacks. *Newman's Bavarian Pretzels* cut out at least the cooked vegetable oils. There are so called "raw food" bars out there such as *Lara Bars* and *Raweos.* I ate these frequently when I was transitioning to a fully raw diet. Although they taste really good, especially the *Raweos*, they always gave me a stomach ache. This is because most of them use "raw" cashews. Raw cashews are not really raw. They are de-shelled through a heating process and this can cause digestive issues. Also, I do not think many of these companies are using soaked or sprouted nuts which again can cause digestive issues. If nuts are sprouted or soaked, the companies will display it on the label. The manufacturers of these products understand the importance and are very proud of what they offer.

Fruit and raw cheese can be eaten as snacks as well. Too much raw cheese with salt can cause constipation but I have not had that experience with no-salt raw cheese.

I drink smoothies, and the lemon/cider honey drink as snacks. It is a good idea to always have raw meats and unsalted raw cheese available in your refrigerator so that when you get hungry, you have something to nibble on.

I have listed the ten things to change to transition to a raw diet and they are listed in no specific order. I recommend reading through all of them carefully to see which ones seem the easiest for you and incorporating the easiest ones first. You may make only one change for several weeks or months before you take the next step and that is ok. Everyone is at a different place with regards to their eating habits. It took me several years to transition to a 100% raw diet. I offer support and consultations if you would like guidance in your transition. Go to my website at www.RawToRadiant.com for contact information and phone numbers.

Closing Words

I am often asked questions like, "What if I really want a cup of coffee?" My response is, "Have a cup of coffee." My goal here was awareness. I am not asking you to completely change your life. You will be amazed at how good you feel when you are eating raw and how badly you feel when you are not. Your transition to raw will just happen. I am presenting this information to you so that you are fully informed and can make conscious choices, whatever those choices are for you at this time in your life.

Sometimes hearing information like what I have presented is very difficult, because accepting what I say to be true means everything you have been told is a "lie", and everything you have been doing and providing for yourself and your family is unhealthy.

For example, in order for me to accept this information, I had to admit I had an addiction to chocolate, coffee and cooked foods.

I remember hearing Maya Angelou speaking once and although I don't remember her exact quote, it went something like this..."Sometimes we do things because we don't know better, but once we know better, we can do better".

Our food is an energy source and we have the choice to put life or death into our bodies. Dead food creates death and **Life Creates Life!** Choose to live!

Section III

Recipes

Basic Green Juice

½ Stalk Celery
½ - 1 large Cucumber or Zucchini
¼ bunch Fresh Parsley

Juice vegetables and then put through a strainer to remove pulp.
Optional: Adding 1 teaspoon fresh raw cow cream (will help bind with toxins and will make the juice taste amazing).

Lemon - Cider Honey Tea/Drink

Juice of ½ Lemon
1 Tablespoon Raw Apple Cider Vinegar
1 Heaping Tablespoon Raw Honey

Warm water just enough so you can put your finger in it without burning it. Add your ingredients listed above and enjoy!

*I also put this same mixture in naturally sparkling spring water for a cooler refreshing drink.

Rob's Coconut Lemonade
Recipe created by Rob Kurtz

8 – 12 oz Fresh Coconut Water/Milk
½ Small Lime, peeled
½ Small Lemon, peeled
1 Heaping Tablespoon Raw Unheated Honey

Blend all ingredients in blender until honey mixed in well. Add 1 cup or more of ice and blend again. Enjoy this delicious, refreshing drink!
Serving size: 2

Note: Use the fresh coconut water from inside the coconut when making coconut cream, not the store bought pasteurized coconut water.

Tropical Smoothie

3 Raw Eggs
1/8 – ¼ Pineapple
1 Tbls Raw Unheated Honey
1 Tbls Coconut Oil and/or Coconut Cream
1 Tbls fresh Raw Cow Cream (optional)
Blend in blender until honey is well mixed.
Add: Frozen Organic Strawberries. Blend and serve.

*I like this smoothie best but you can use any kind of fruit you like. The frozen berries give it that thick frosty desert-like taste. If no frozen fruit is available, use ice to thicken it up.

Try:
Mango & Strawberry
Pineapple & Mango
Banana & Blueberry

Orange Smoothie
I use this one for the onset of illness

2-3 Raw Eggs
1 Tablespoon Raw Unheated Honey
Juice of 3-4 fresh Organic Oranges

Blend all ingredients in blender until honey is mixed in well. Add equal amount of ice and blend in blender until thick and frosty.

*My daughter and I have these and only these at the onset of a cold/flu or fever, get plenty of rest and the detoxification process only lasts 24 hours...every time!

<u>Wild Salmon & Shrimp Ceviche'</u>

Fresh Wild Salmon ½ lb
Raw Shrimp ½ lb
Organic Limes

<u>Sauce:</u>
Tomatoes – ¼ quart cherry, chopped
Jalapeno pepper – ½ -1 finely diced
Red Onion – equal portion to jalapeno, finely diced
Ginger – 1 ½ tsp, finely diced
Cilantro – ½ bunch
Raw Apple Cider Vinegar – equal amount to olive oil
(approximately 1/3 – ½ cup)
Virgin or Extra Virgin Olive Oil – equal amount to vinegar
(approximately 1/3 – ½ cup)
Raw, Unheated Honey – 1 Tablespoon
Avocado – ½ to 1, cut into chunks

Cut up fish into small pieces (1/2 inch) and marinate in lime juice. Let sit in refrigerator while you are making the sauce. Ok to let marinate a few hours or overnight.
Chop jalapeno, red onion, ginger, tomato and cilantro and place into bowl. You can never have too much cilantro!
Pour equal amounts raw apple cider vinegar & olive oil...just enough to cover top of ingredients.
Add raw honey and mix well.
Cut avocado into chunks and mix in last so it does not get mushy. I like large chunks of avocado & tomato.
Pour lime juice off of fish and place fish into serving bowl.
Mix sauce into fish.
For smaller appetizer portions, serve in empty avocado halves.

Serves 1-2, 3-5 appetizer portions
Everyone loves this dish. This is a great recipe for those starting a raw diet.

Filet Appetizer

Freshly cut Filet Steak (Beef Tenderloin)
1 Medium Tomato
Raw Unsalted Cheese
Fresh Basil

Slice filet, tomato and raw cheese into thin strips
Layer the following on top of one another:
>   Tomato slice
>   Raw sliced filet
>   Raw cheese
>   Small piece of basil

This is wonderful as an appetizer or as a way to eat the entire steak. I highly recommend this recipe for beginners and anyone squeamish about eating raw red meats.

Serves 1 as a meal and 4 as appetizers.

*You can also slice filet into thin strips and eat with guacamole and raw cheese.

Buffalo Tartar

1 lb - Ground Buffalo
¼ quart Cherry Tomatoes – chopped
½ - 1 Jalapeno pepper – diced
Red Onion – equal to jalapeno, diced
1 tsp Fresh Ginger – diced
4 Fresh Basil Leaves – chopped
¼ - 1/3 cup Raw Apple Cider Vinegar
¼ - 1/3 cup Virgin or Extra Virgin Olive Oil
1 Tablespoon Raw Unheated Honey
½ to 1 Avocado

Place ground buffalo in bowl.
<u>Sauce:</u>
Put tomato, jalapeno, red onion, ginger and basil into separate bowl.
Pour in equal amounts olive oil and apple cider vinegar; enough to almost cover vegetables.
Add raw honey and mix well.
Add avocado into sauce last.
Mix sauce into beef and serve.
You can use circular molds to form.
Garnish with fresh tomato and avocado slices

Kathleen's Meat Loaf:
Recipe created by Kathleen Wanatowicz

1 pound Ground Beef (hormone & antibiotic free)
1 tsp Cumin Spice
1 raw egg
1 tsp Rosemary
1 tsp. Tarragon
Diced celery to taste
½ dried shallot

Combine all ingredients in a bowl. Roll into small bite size balls (about the size of a quarter).

Serve with sides of: Tomatoes, Raw Pumpkin seeds & Freshly Diced Ginger.

Beginner Chicken

Cut a whole boneless, skinless chicken breast into small pieces and put in a bowl. Cover the chicken with enough fresh lemon juice to cover the top. Let marinade for 1 hour to overnight (lemon and lime kill bacteria). While marinating, cut the following into little pieces:

Half a Jalapeno Pepper
¼ inch slice of a Red Onion
¼ inch slice of Tomato
Raw Unsalted Cheese
Fresh Basil
½ - 1 Avocado

Drain lemon off of chicken and place in serving bowl.
In separate bowl make sauce with tomato, jalapeno, red onion, ginger and basil.
Pour in equal amounts olive oil and apple cider vinegar, enough to almost cover vegetables.
Add raw honey and mix well.
Add avocado into sauce last.
Mix sauce into chicken and serve.

Pour 1/8 cup of raw apple cider vinegar over chicken. Add 1/8 cup virgin olive oil to chicken. Add ingredients you cut up. Mix well. Add 2-3 heaping tablespoons raw unheated honey. Mix well and enjoy.

Avocado Custard
Recipe created by Alecia Evans

2 Raw Eggs
1 Avocado
½ Medium Tomato (optional)
3 Tablespoons Raw Unsalted Butter
1 Tablespoon Coconut Cream
1 -2 Tablespoons Raw Unheated Honey (to taste)

Put all ingredients in blender and blend until creamy.
Serves 1-2.

Note: Some people have problems digesting avocados and others have no problem with them. Test it out and see how your body does. You can cut the amount of avocado in half, if needed.

Peach Ice Cream

1 Raw Egg
¼ - 1/3 qt Fresh Raw Cow Cream
1 Heaping Tablespoon Raw Unheated Honey
1 – 2 Peeled Fresh Organic Peaches

Mix ingredients in blender and place in ice cream maker.
If you are using frozen peaches, make sure to mix egg, cream
and honey first so honey can blend into mixture well. Then,
add frozen fruit.
Serving size: 2-3

Banana Ginger Ice Cream

1 Raw Egg
¼ - 1/3 qt Fresh Raw Cow Cream
1 Heaping Tablespoon Raw Unheated Honey
1 Peeled Organic Banana
1 tsp Fresh Ginger Juice (make in a juicer)

Mix ingredients in blender and place in ice cream maker.
Serving size: 2-3

Natashia's Banana Cream Pie
Recipe created by Natashia Cohen

Crust: Nut Butter Recipe from "*The Recipe for Living Without Disease*", Aajonus Vonderplanitz
2 – 4 oz Raw Pecans or Walnuts
4 – 8 Tablespoons Raw Unsalted Butter – room temperature
1 – 2 Raw Eggs
1 ½ - 2 Tablespoons Raw Honey

•   Blenderize nuts in an 8 or 12 oz canning jar on high speed until they are flour. Add remaining ingredients and stir. Blenderize on medium speed for 20 – 25 seconds, until smooth.

Banana Filling:
Ripe bananas mashed
Raw Honey
Mix a small amount (to taste) of honey in with the mashed bananas.

Topping:
Raw Cream
Raw Honey
•   Mix a small amount of honey (to taste) with the cream and whip with a hand mixer until firm.

Layer as follows: Crust, filling and topping.
Make small individual servings or one large serving.
Serve immediately or refrigerate for ½ to 1 hour before serving.

Coconut Balls

2 Cups Coconut Meat/Pulp (left over from making coconut
cream in the juicer)
¼ cup Walnuts, finely chopped
3 Eggs
3 Tablespoons Raw Honey

Place coconut meat in bowl. In an 8 oz. canning jar with a
blender blade (see equipment/blender), blend walnuts until
finely chopped and add to coconut. Blend eggs and honey
together and add to coconut mixture. Mix in well. Make balls
about the size of a nickel and place on a tray. Refrigerate for
two hours. Best served cold out of the refrigerator.
Makes approximately 30 coconut balls.

References

"We Want To Live", Aajonus Vonderplanitz, 2005 edition

"The Recipe For Living Without Disease", Aajonus Vonderplanitz, 2002

"Enzyme Nutrition: The Food Enzyme Concept", Dr. Edward Howell, 1985

"Home Safe Home", Debra Lynn Dadd, 1997

"The Real Truth About Vitamins & Antioxidants", Health Science Series #5, 1997 Judith A. DeCava, MS, LNC

"Food Is Your Best Medicine", Henry G. Bieler, MD, twelfth printing, April 1992

"Diet, Nutrition, and Cancer", Committee on Diet, Nutrition and Cancer. Assembly of Life Sciences. National Research Council, 1982

"Health: The Only Immunity", Ian Sinclair, 1995

"Notes on Microbial Infection for Medical Physicists", Dr. John Heritage, of the School of Biochemistry and Molecular Biology at the University of Leeds.

"Sick and Tired", Dr. Robert Young, 2001

"Pasteur or Beauchamp?", E. Douglas Hume (C.W. Daniel Co. 1923, Reprint 1989, Health Research.

"Conscious Eating", Gabriel Cousins, 2000

"Rethinking Chlorinated Tap Water", Article by Dr. Zoltan P. Rona, MD, MSc

"Early Death comes From Drinking Distilled Water", article by Zoltan P. Rona, MD, MSc

"Dangers of Refined Sugar", article by Dr. William Coda Martin, 1/08/2003

"Patient Heal Thyself", Jordan S. Rubin, N.M.D, C.N.C, 2003

"Sugar Blues", William Duffy, 1975

"Honey as a Dressing for Wounds, Burns, and Ulcers: A Brief Review of Clinical Reports and Experimental Studies", Published in Primary Intention Vol. 6, no. 4, December 1998, P.C. Molan, B.Sc. Ph.D., Honey Research Unit, Department of Biological Sciences, University of Waikato, Hamilton, New Zealand.

"76 Ways Sugar Can Ruin Your Health", article by Dr. Joseph Mercola on <u>Mercola.com</u> and contributed by Nancy Appleton, Ph.D, author of the book, *"Lick The Sugar Habit"*.

"A Faulty Medical Model: The Germ Theory", article without reference to author, <u>www.life-enthusiast.com</u>

"Adventures in Diet" a series of articles from Harpers Magazine November 1935 to January 1936 by Vilhjalmur Stefansson
"Anthropological Research Reveals Human Dietary Requirements for Optimal Health", article by H Leon Abrams, Jr., MA EDS, Journal of Applied Nutrition, 1982, 16:1:38-45

Heterocyclic Amines: Occurrence and Prevention in Cooked Food, Saida Robbana-Barnat,[1] Maurice Rabache,[2] Emmanuelle Rialland,[2] and Jacques Fradin[1] , Environmental Health

Perspectives, Vol. 104, Number 3, March 1996. [1]Institut de Médecine Environnementale, 75014 Paris, France; [2]Conservatoire National des Arts et Métiers, Equipe Génie Biologique, 75

Sinha R, Rothman N, Brown ED, Salmon C, Kinze M, Swanson A, Rossi S, Mark S, Levander O, Felton J. High concentration of the carcinogen 2-amino-1-methyl-6-phenylimidazo[4,5-b]pyridine (PhIP) occur in chicken but are dependent on the cooking method. Cancer Res 55:516-4519 (1995). 003 Paris, France

"Can we prevent and cure most diseases by nutrition?" paper written by D. Paul Cohen, president of the Cohen Independent Research Group, a Wall Street research firm, after an interview with Dr. Aajonus Vonderplanitz.

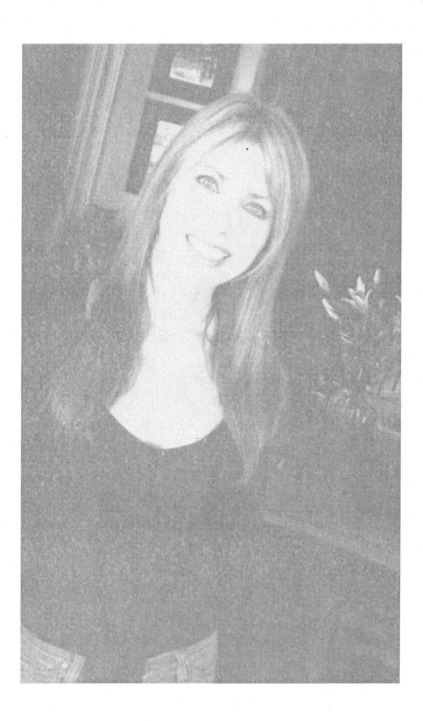

About The Author

Kim Cohen began studying nutrition out of necessity when her daughter Sedona was born with severe food allergies. Her journeys lead her down several alternative paths. In 2001, Kim created *Idella's Natural Gourmet*, an organic cookie company that made cookies for people with food allergies and sensitivities. About the same time, she began studying raw food nutrition, learning how the cooking process negatively affects nutrition and health.

During her raw foods education, she learned the truth of what cooked vegetable oils do in the body and felt she could no longer consciously sell her baked cookies. She closed the doors of *Idella's;* but as one door closed, another opened and Kim became a nutritional consultant, counseling people on the health benefits of raw foods. A member of the American Association of Nutritional Consultants, she currently travels the country conducting lectures and workshops to both groups and individuals on the subject of nutrition, food preparation and how to integrate raw life-giving foods into their current diet and lifestyle.

Index

A

Acryl amides, 9,10
Acute disease, 14
Advanced Glycation End Products, 9
Allergies, 40
Alzheimer's, v, 14
Anemia, 15
Arthritis, 14
Asthma, 40
Atherosclerosis, v
Autism, vi
Avocado custard, 100

B

Bacteria, 10, 15, 17, 18, 19, 20, 23, 40
Banana ginger ice cream, 101
Basic green juice, 91
Beauchamp, Antoine, 21, 23
Beginner chicken, 99
Bieler, Henry, 14
Blenders, 72
    Blendtech, 73
    Total Blender, 73
    Vitamix, 73
Brittle bones, 7

C

Cancer, 15, 16, 17
Canning jars, 73
Carcinogenic, 9
Cause of disease, 3
Chemicals, 67, 68
Childhood illness, 14

Chronic disease, 14
Citrus juicer, 72
Cold, 15, 16
Colonics, 45
Cooking
    Carbohydrates, 9
    Fats, 7
    Fruits/vegetables, 11, 34
    Meats, 10

D

Dairy,
    Raw, 30, 31, 32
DeCava, Judith, 49
Deficiencies, 13
Degenerative disease, 9, 39
Dehydrating, 63
Detoxification, 13, 15, 20
Diabetes, v, 14
Diarrhea, 13
Digestion, 45
Digestive enzymes, 8
DNA, 4
Dodd, Debra Lynn, 64, 68

E

Eating out, 57
Edible oils, 8
Elimination, 45
Enderlein, Gunther, 21, 23
Endobionts, 21, 22
Enzyme inhibitors, 55
Enzymes, 6,35,53,54
    Digestive, 8, 53, 54
    Food, 53, 54
    Metabolic, 53, 54
Equipment, 71

Expeller pressing, 8

F

Fats,
    Cooked, 7
    Raw, 30, 32
Fibromyalgia, 14
Filet appetizer, 96
Flu, 15
Food combining, 43
Fruits
    Raw, 34

G

Germ theory, 21
Glycotoxins, 9
Green Star juicer, 71

H

Heart disease, v
Heptane, 8
Herbivores, 27
Heritage, John, 22
Heterocyclic amines, 10
Hexane, 8
High meat, 16
Honey, raw, 35, 36, 37
    Benefits, 36, 37

I

Ice cream makers
    Donvier, 72
Integration, 75
Ionic charge, 30
Iridology, 47

J

Juicers, 71
    Citrus, 72
    Green Star, 71
Juices
    Bottled, 77
    Vegetable, 33, 75, 76

L

Lemon cider tea, 92
Lifestyle changes, 67

M

Malnutrition, 3, 4
Meat eaters, 25
Meats,
    Cooked, 10
    Raw, 32
Meat loaf, 98
Microzyma, 22
Mold, 15, 19, 23,
Monomorphic, 21
Mutagens, 4, 9, 10
Myelin, 31, 37, 38

N

Natashia's banana cream pie, 97
National Cancer Institute, 3
National Research Council, 3, 9, 10
Negative ionic charge, 30
Nuts,
    Raw, 34

O

Obesity, vi
Orange smoothie, 94
Organ density, 62
Osteoporosis, 7, 15, 40

P

Parasites, 15, 19, 23
Parkinson's, 15
Pasteur, Louis, 21, 22, 23, 24
Pasteurized, 7, 8, 11
Peach ice cream, 101
Phytonutrients, 6, 11
Pleomorphic, 21
Positive ionic charge, 30
Pottenger, Frances, 7, 39
Probiotics, 40
Price, Weston, 39

R

Raw dairy, 30, 31, 32
Raw fats, 30
Raw foods, 29, 47
Raw foods diet, 1
Raw fruits, 34
Raw honey, 35
Raw integration, 75
Raw meats, 32
Raw nuts, 34
Raw vegetables, 33
Recipes
  Avocado custard, 100
  Banana ginger ice cream, 101
  Basic green juice, 91
  Beginner chicken, 99
  Buffalo tartar, 97
  Coconut balls, 103
  Filet appetizer, 96
  Lemon cider tea, 92
  Meat loaf, 98
  Natashia's banana cream pie, 102
  Orange smoothie, 94
  Peach ice cream, 101
  Rob's lemonade, 93
  Tropical smoothie, 93
  Wild salmon & shrimp ceviche, 95
Rob's lemonade, 93

S

Salmonella, 17
Sinclair, Ian, 14
Solvent extraction, 8
Soy, 18
Spices, 37
Statistics
  Atherosclerosis, v
  Autism, vi
  Cancer, v
  Heart disease, v
  Obesity, vi
Stefansson, Vilhjalmur, 40
Stenosis, 7
Storage containers, 73
Sugar, 82, 83
Supplements, 49

Sushi, 18, 78, 79, 80

T

Terramin clay, 64, 71, 84, 91
Toxemia, 3, 4, 13
Travel blender/juicer, 72
Tropical smoothie, 90

U

Ulcers, 14
Unpasteurized, 7, 8
Unrefined oils, 8

V

Vegan, 1
Vegetables,
  Cooked, 11
  Raw, 33
Vegetarians, 25
Viruses, 15, 16, 17, 18
Vitamins, 11, 49
  Fractionated, 49
  Synthetic, 49, 50
  Whole food, 49, 50
Vonderplanitz, Aajonus, 22, 32, 79

W

Water, 63
  Distilled, 66
  Natural sparkling, 63
  Public, 64, 65
  Spring, 63
  Tap, 64, 65
  Toxins in, 65
  Well, 64
Weight, 61
Wild salmon & shrimp ceviche, 95

Y

Young, Robert, 21

Receive 20% off additional copies of:

Raw To Radiant:
The Secrets To A Long Life Of Radiant Health Through Raw Foods

Purchase 10 or more books and receive 20% off the cover price. ***Raw To Radiant*** makes great gifts for family and friends.
You must call us directly for this special offer:

970-920-2142

Products Order Form

Bill To:
Name:_____
Address:_____
City:_____ State:_____
Zip:_____ Phone:_____

Ship To:
Name:_____
Address:_____
City:_____ State:_____
Zip:_____ Phone:_____

Qty	Description	Size	Cost	Total
_____	Raw Unheated **Honey**	Half Gallon	$36.00	_____
_____	Raw Unheated **Honey**	Gallon	$51.00	_____
_____	Raw Unheated **Coconut Oil**	Pint (16oz)	$15.95	_____
_____	Raw Unheated **Coconut Oil**	Quart (32oz)	$20.95	_____
_____	Raw Unheated **Coconut Oil**	1/2 Gallon (64 oz)	$36.95	_____
_____	**Terramin** Clay	1 lb	$16.95	_____
_____	Terramin Clay	2 lb	$29.95	_____
_____	**Pure Aussie** Sea Minerals	8 oz	$15.00	_____
_____	Pure Aussie *Supa Boost*	8 oz	$45.00	_____
_____	Pure Aussie *Hawthorne*	8 oz	$45.00	_____
_____	Pure Aussie *Stinging Nettle*	8 oz	$45.00	_____
_____	Pure Aussie *CPRA* therapeutic cream		$20.00	_____
_____	Pure Aussie *Nabolji* face & neck cream		$15.00	_____
_____	**Green Star** Juicer	**1000 model**	$379.00	_____
_____	Green Star Juicer	2000 model	$399.00	_____
_____	**Bullet** Travel Juicer/Blender		$49.95	_____
_____	Blendtech **Total Blender**	Black/White	$399.00	_____
_____	Donvier **Ice Cream Maker**		$53.00	_____
_____	Star Popsicle Mold	Push Up Style	$19.95	_____
_____	Rocket Popsicle Mold		$14.95	_____
_____	Book - *"Raw To Radiant"*		$19.95	_____
_____	Book - *"We Want To Live"*		$29.95	_____
_____	Book - *"Recipes for Living Without Disease"*		$29.95	_____
_____	Book - *"Home Safe Home"*		$19.95	_____
_____	Leaf People Skin Care - starter	**Transformation**	$35.00	_____
_____	Leaf People Skin Care - starter	**Daily Rejuvinate**	$30.00	_____
_____	Leaf People Skin Care - starter	**Combination**	$30.00	_____
_____	Leaf People Himilayan Bath Salts		$20.00	_____

Sub Total: _____
CO Sales Tax 2.9%: _____
TOTAL: _____

_____Check payable to: *Raw to Radiant*   _____Credit Card
Visa____   Master Card_____   Discover_____   Am Express_____
Name On Card: _____
Billing Address:_____
City: _____ State: _____ Zip: _____
Billing Phone: _____ E-Mail: _____
Card Number:_____ exp:_____ 3 digit code:_____

Fax to: 775-514-0532 or Mail to: PO Box 1612 Aspen, CO 81612

Products Order Form

Bill To: **Ship To:**

Name:_____   Name:_____

Address:_____   Address:_____

City:_____ State:_____   City:_____ State:_____

Zip:_____ Phone:_____   Zip:_____ Phone:_____

Qty	Description	Size	Cost	Total
_____	Raw Unheated **Honey**	Half Gallon	$36.00	
_____	Raw Unheated **Honey**	Gallon	$51.00	
_____	Raw Unheated **Coconut Oil**	Pint (16oz)	$15.95	
_____	Raw Unheated **Coconut Oil**	Quart (32oz)	$20.95	
_____	Raw Unheated **Coconut Oil**	1/2 Gallon (64 oz)	$36.95	
_____	**Terramin** Clay	1 lb	$16.95	
_____	Terramin Clay	2 lb	$29.95	
_____	**Pure Aussie** Sea Minerals	8 oz	$15.00	
_____	Pure Aussie *Supa Boost*	8 oz	$45.00	
_____	Pure Aussie *Hawthorne*	8 oz	$45.00	
_____	Pure Aussie *Stinging Nettle*	8 oz	$45.00	
_____	Pure Aussie *CPRA* therapeutic cream		$20.00	
_____	Pure Aussie *Nabolji* face & neck cream		$15.00	
_____	**Green Star** Juicer	**1000 model**	$379.00	
_____	Green Star Juicer	2000 model	$399.00	
_____	**Bullet** Travel Juicer/Blender		$49.95	
_____	Blendtech **Total Blender**	Black/White	$399.00	
_____	Donvier **Ice Cream Maker**		$53.00	
_____	Star Popsicle Mold	Push Up Style	$19.95	
_____	Rocket Popsicle Mold		$14.95	
_____	Book - "*Raw To Radiant*"		$19.95	
_____	Book - "*We Want To Live*"		$29.95	
_____	Book -"*Recipes for Living Without Disease*"		$29.95	
_____	Book -"*Home Safe Home*"		$19.95	
_____	Leaf People Skin Care - starter	**Transformation**	$35.00	
_____	Leaf People Skin Care - starter	**Daily Rejuvinate**	$30.00	
_____	Leaf People Skin Care - starter	**Combination**	$30.00	
_____	Leaf People Himilayan Bath Salts		$20.00	

Sub Total: _____

CO Sales Tax 2.9%: _____

TOTAL: _____

_____Check payable to: *Raw to Radiant*   _____Credit Card

Visa_____   Master Card_____   Discover_____   Am Express_____

Name On Card: _____

Billing Address:_____

City: _____ State: _____ Zip: _____

Billing Phone: _____ E-Mail: _____

Card Number:_____ exp:_____ 3 digit code:_____

Fax to: 775-514-0532 or Mail to: PO Box 1612 Aspen, CO 81612

Raw To Radiant Institute
PO Box 1612
Aspen, CO 81612
970-920-2142 phone
775-514-0532 fax

www.RawToRadiant.com
Kim@RawToRadiant.com